GETTING OLD: DEAL
WITH IT

LEE JANOGLY

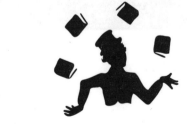

MENSCH PUBLISHING

Mensch Publishing
51 Northchurch Road, London N1 4EE, United Kingdom

First published in Great Britain 2020

A catalogue record for this book is available from the British Library

ISBN: PB: 978-1-912914-03-6; eBook: 978-1-912914-04-3

2 4 6 8 10 9 7 5 3 1

Typeset by Newgen KnowledgeWorks Pvt. Ltd., Chennai, India
Printed and bound in Great Britain by CPI Group (UK) Ltd, Croydon CR0 4YY

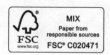

For my beloved grandchildren
Jack, Gabs, Levi, Gigi, Ava, Rosa and Talia
This will happen to you one day!

In memory of Avril Norden
1921–2018
who grew old so gracefully

CONTENTS

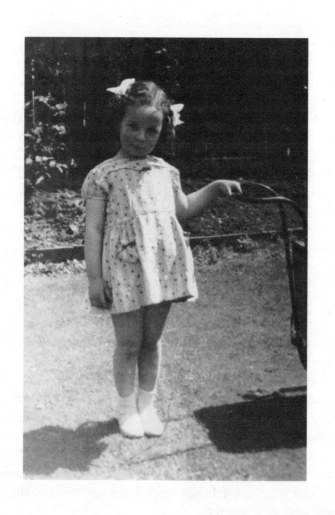

PROLOGUE

1943

I am four years old and, as you can see in the picture, I am wearing my new white shoes which I mustn't get dirty. I was born with frizzy, unmanageable hair which could only be tamed by my mummy winding sections of wet hair round her finger and dropping each one into a large sausage curl, which she would tie into bunches with ribbons. My mummy is very old. I know this because when she sits on a chair her feet touch the floor.

My sister has just been born. She is called 'the baby' and I don't like her. Mummy said do you want to kiss the baby and I said no. I hope they send her back.

Everyone around me is talking about the WAR. My daddy is in charge of that because he is the 'WAR-den' and has to wear an itchy brown uniform. My daddy is very old. I know this because he has to scrape the hair off his face every morning.

Sometimes there is a very loud noise which means the naughty men are going to fly over in their aeroplanes and make the bangs. They are called The Nasties. When that happens my daddy shouts, 'come on, come on, hurry up' and everyone stops what they are doing and we all run into a deep cave in the garden – I think it's called an airing shoulder – until the bangs stop. Then my daddy calls 'all clear' and we come out.

Most days, though, I go to school. My mummy walks me there and on the way we pass some men from another country called American-Air-Base. One of the men is tall with a silly haircut which makes his head flat. He is very old and waits for mummy and me to pass by every day and we stop for a chat. I think he is a friend of Mummy's because she does that funny smiley thing and looks up at him through her eyelashes. His name is Howie and he gives her bars of chocolate and chewing gum. Mummy kisses him to say thank you. Her kisses last a long time so he must give her lots of chewing gum. Then Mummy says to me, 'Say goodbye to Howie,' and I try to look up at him through my eyelashes like she does, but she just says to me 'What's the matter, do you feel sick?'

I don't like school at all and cry every day. I thought if I cried loud enough mummy would take me home but she doesn't, she just waits by the door. I keep looking round to see if she is still there because I want to stay with her and not get evacuumed like the children next door, but she must have slipped off while I was playing with plasticine, which isn't fair. We learned a song in a foreign language which goes 'Mairzy doats and dozy doats and liddle lamzy divey, a kiddley divey too wooden you.'

At break time we play ball and I like that, though I do feel sorry for someone called Hitler that people sing a song about, because we have lots of balls and he only has one.

I hope when the war is finished I won't have to go to school any more. But my daddy said when it's all over he will buy me a bicycle and I can also have a banana. I don't know how to ride a banana but I'm sure I'll soon learn.

I suppose I will be very old one day. I'll know this because when I sit on a chair my feet will touch the floor.

Fast forward 76 years...

I

ARE YOU OLD?

Have you ever stood behind an old, old person at the checkout in a supermarket? She watches as the cashier helpfully packs her shopping for her, whilst chatting happily about the weather and how it affects her arthritis. Once her purchases are safely in her tartan wheelie bag she stands there expectantly until it dawns on her: Oh yes, she has to pay for it! There's a surprise. Only then does she dive into her cavernous bag to find her purse – her Clubcard – rummage, rummage, now where is it? It should be – maybe it's in the zippered compartment – oh, what have we here, some money-off coupons! Are these still valid? No dear, they expired three months ago, and these are for Boots and this is Tesco. Really? Oh, what a shame. She peers at the display then counts out her coins to the exact penny, while you jiggle and fume with irritation. Don't. One day that will probably be you.

Or me. I have to confess I'm the one holding up the queue at the cinema in front of the machine, trying to extract my pre-ordered tickets which it is reluctant to part with, or give me back my credit card. Or did I insert my travel card by mistake? Maybe. That is also me calling loudly for a human assistant at the self-service checkout in the super-market to try and quell the infernal bleating of the voice insisting that 'there is an unidentified object in the bagging area.' CAN I GET SOME HELP HERE? What? Oh, it's my umbrella. Sorry.

Me, old? Nah.

You may have noticed another sign. Whenever you are talking to an older person, whatever the subject, she will eventually contrive to inject her age into the conversation, whether it's relevant or not. 'Yes, airports are a nightmare today, you have to walk for miles to get to the gate, but I can manage even though (pause for maximum effect) I'm 73, you know.' The pride with which they say this leaves you no choice but to stagger back in amazement and tell them it's not possible as they look no older than 40. You lie.

It seems that everyone wants to *be* the oldest and *look* the youngest. They get so used to the faux surprised and complimentary comments about how young they look that eventually, when asked their age, they craftily add a year, such as 'Next year I'll be 74.' No! Really?!

The obvious lesson to be learned here is never ask anyone to guess your age. They may get it right! 'I don't look 73, do I?' (Not anymore!)

I think we're all deluded about our age to a certain extent depending on our mood or whether we had a good night's sleep. I know that sometimes I can look in the mirror and think, 'You know what, you don't look bad.' Other times, particularly after a late night which included some sugary dessert followed by a bar of Cadbury's finest, the same mirror shows a raddled, puffy old hag with lines and wrinkles that definitely weren't there the day before. Some mirrors are just like that.

In my opinion age falls roughly into the following categories:

Up to 20 = very young
20 – 35 = young and lovely
35 – 50 = lovely
50 – 70 = middle-aged
70 – 80 = mature and wise
80 – 90 = old
90 – 100 = ancient
100+ = you've overstayed your welcome, time to leave
the party

If, like me, you were born in the 1930s or 40s I often wonder how we managed to reach adulthood relatively intact. I remember as a child of eight or nine going off on my bike after breakfast to meet my friends during the school holidays, and not coming home until teatime. As long as I eventually turned up, my mother didn't seem concerned at all. At the local park or wherever I was, I don't remember being accosted by anyone unpleasant, nor were there gangs roaming around looking for someone to mug or stab. I can't imagine a child today being allowed to roam free in that way.

Being old now, though, does have its advantages: there is the Freedom Pass allowing you free or reduced travel around the UK, cheaper cinema seats, people stand up to offer you a seat on the tube – well, they do when I glare at them – and you save a fortune on Tampax. I guess that's it as far as practical things are concerned.

Mentally, you get to a stage where other people's opinions just brush off you. Very few people reach an advanced age without experiencing a few knocks along the way and this leads to a realisation of what is important in life and what isn't. You make your choices and take responsibility for them and if other people don't like them, well, that's tough!

However, being old doesn't mean you have to 'think' old. If you think of yourself as old, you will appear to others that way and they will treat you accordingly. We all know people who seem to be decrepit at 30 and others who are still spritely in their nineties. I remember hosting a tea party for my mother's 90th birthday and inviting a close friend of hers aged 97. She declined the invitation as she was flying to Spain that weekend to take part in a chess tournament.

If you aren't in good health it's very hard to think young, although believing yourself to be in better than normal condition for your age is typical of healthy people in general. People who think young compare themselves with others of the same age in a more positive light.

It's difficult *not* to think of yourself as old when you are constantly reminded of it by the unconscious attitudes of other people. Compliments always come with a caveat: 'She looks amazing *for her age*'; 'He *still* does the Times crossword every day!' Ah, the 'still' word. I'm a fitness instructor and people I haven't seen for a while say to me, 'are you still teaching?' Yeah! Are you still breathing?!

How do *you* see yourself? Do you have an 'old' attitude? When did you last say:

'I have to get my grandson to record programmes for me on the TV.'

'I'm too nervous to use a computer.'

'I only bought a mobile so I could use pay-by-phone to park the bloody car.'

'What happened to directory enquiries?'

'I thought a mouse was a rodent, an apple was a fruit,
    and a cloud was an overcast day!'

Come on, we've all done it, that sudden realisation that
we are not as young as we once were. They say you know
you're old when your children talk to each other in front of
you and spell out certain words.

You can't help being old, it's not a crime. As Mark Twain
said: 'Age is an issue of mind over matter. If you don't mind,
it doesn't matter.' But I'm afraid in our society, ageism
against older people is still alive and kicking. Ageism is
what happens when people are defined not by their personality, individuality or beliefs but by their age. Check out
some of the misconceptions about old people.

MYTH NO. 1. OLD PEOPLE ARE SLOW-MINDED

Not so. There may be some cognitive changes as you age
but this just means older people may perform better in certain areas of intelligence and not so well in others. Maybe
we do find it difficult to add up a series of numbers in our
heads, but we adapt to the slowing of memory by making
lists and altering our approach to retaining information.
Certain mental capabilities that depend very much on
accumulated experience and knowledge, like dealing with
people in authority and increasing one's vocabulary, clearly
get better over time.

It's acknowledged by most motoring organisations that
older people have fewer accidents than youngsters hot-
rodding it along the motorways, in spite of Prince Philip
somersaulting his car at the age of 97. Luckily no one was
seriously hurt. Usually, however, older drivers are very

aware that their reactions may be a bit slower, so they drive more cautiously and with greater care on the road. Personally, I hate driving on busy main roads and as for motorways – forget it!

MYTH NO. 2. OLD PEOPLE ALL HAVE SIMILAR TRAITS

Again, not so. Research has shown that as we age, we become more differentiated, more individualised and less like one another. None of us gets older in exactly the same way and each of us ages at a different rate. Anyone who has been to a class reunion can verify that there are some former classmates who seem to have turned into their mothers while others look just like us.

MYTH NO. 3. OLD PEOPLE ARE WEAK AND FRAIL

Maybe some people are but not at the health centre that I go to. There are about thirty treadmills and cross-trainers in the gym and often there is a spritely, white-haired person slogging away on each one. Another few have personal trainers guiding them to lift weights safely. I prefer the aerobic classes to music (preferably Motown) which, again, are populated by many older people and consist of continuous movement for nearly an hour. This class is not for weaklings!

Having said that, there is a marked acceleration of frailty in someone who has had a serious fall – or as we refer to it 'an unplanned appointment with the pavement.' This can happen so easily and is sudden and shocking. One minute you are walking along the street quite normally, the next you're sprawled on the ground, shopping and handbag flying in all directions. The embarrassment is compounded by kindly people rushing to help you and made worse if an ambulance has to be called.

If the fall results in a fractured wrist or femur head requiring the dreaded hip replacement, this could change your mindset as to how you see yourself as you are terrified it will happen again. You may start to walk more gingerly rather than striding out and once you succumb to using a stick, this cements your vision of yourself as an old person.

Problems can arise however if you get used to the reassurance of the stick even when you're fully recovered. This is a personal decision of course but maybe a few sessions of intense physiotherapy or a personal trainer would give you back your confidence to dispense with the stick when the time is right.

Becoming frail after a hip replacement doesn't necessarily follow though. My mother had advanced dementia when she suffered a fall in her nursing home, breaking her hip. She was taken to hospital where the surgeon patiently explained to her what the ensuing operation entailed. She gazed at him intently as he spoke and when he had finished she looked at me and said, 'Isn't he handsome!' (he was) – clearly not understanding a word he said.

Because of her dementia, after the operation she walked perfectly normally, not realising that she had had anything done. The staff were amazed when at her discharge, three days later, she walked down the steps to the car without a thought.

MYTH NO. 4. YOU CAN'T TEACH AN OLD DOG NEW TRICKS

Yes, you can. This old dog is teaching herself to play the piano and although I have never mastered the art of reading music, I can knock out a cool boogie-woogie riff to my immense satisfaction. I spoke to a huge number of older women while I was researching this book and so many of them are taking courses in writing, painting, architecture appreciation, learning a new language etc. Automatically assuming that learning and creativity inevitably decline with ageing is inaccurate and pessimistic. We are not all sitting at home knitting covers for our hot water bottles!

MYTH NO. 5. OLD PEOPLE ARE FORGETFUL

Sometimes – but so are young people. When I ask my son to do something, his automatic response is 'remind me later' or 'text me when I'm at the office.' (No – make a note, boy, like now!) Most minor forgetfulness is completely normal and inconsequential. Moreover, a *significant* loss of memory represents a disease and is therefore *not* normal ageing. Losing your keys is normal. Finding them in the fridge is not normal. Most people over 85 have completely normal cognitive function.

MYTH NO. 6. AGEING MAKES YOU UNABLE TO ADAPT TO NEW SITUATIONS

Older people not only can adapt to new situations, they have to! More and more companies and services insist that you deal with them online. Banks are reluctant to send out statements and prefer you to download them. Marks & Spencer have removed the post boxes from inside their stores which allowed people to pay their credit card bill by cheque. Now you have to set up a direct debit or post the blasted thing!

A lot of us seniors have cottoned on to shopping online, though, *and* are adept at sending the goods back again! The trouble is, for some, this means you never have to leave the house. And the trouble with that is, often you don't. In many cases this encourages a sedentary lifestyle where it's easier to have groceries delivered rather than push a trolley round a supermarket, so you sit around eating Hobnobs and watching TV.

MYTH NO. 7. OLD PEOPLE ARE UNPRODUCTIVE

There is an assumption that people over 70 are viewed as contributing little to the economy and being a 'burden on health services.' Such views are expressed and perpetuated frequently in the media.

Though retired people may have left the workforce, they are hardly unproductive. Everyone I know who has grandchildren steps in and cares for them on occasions while their parents work, sometimes for days at a time. I love having mine during the school holidays especially now that they are teenagers and we can enjoy the theatre and films, when I can afford it. Retired people also contribute countless hours to volunteering, which makes an enormous impact on society.

The literary editor, Diana Athill, who died in 2019 aged 101, kept working until she was 75 then became an author in her own right in her 80s. She said she was surprised at how much she enjoyed being old but admitted she had been lucky in having good health. Even so, as she put it, 'one does eventually go off the boil, but you shouldn't take the pan off the hob too early.'

MYTH NO. 8. OLD PEOPLE DON'T UNDERSTAND MODERN TEACHING METHODS

I think this is not so much a myth as a reluctance on the part of my generation to move with the times. Certainly, as I watched my 10-year-old granddaughter complete her homework on the nth term before moving on to non-verbal reasoning I hadn't a clue what she was doing.

My friends and I are more concerned with the political slant that is being introduced into many subjects and the curtailment of free expression in favour of rigid adherence to guidelines. A suggestion to enhance an essay being written by another 14-year-old granddaughter (I have five granddaughters and two grandsons) was met with, 'No, that's not what we were told. I'll get a lower grade if I put that.'

Employers despair when taking on university graduates who seem to have a limited knowledge of grammar and spelling. On several occasions, when I have thanked someone for a service, the emailed response of 'Your welcome' seems to be acceptably correct by even the highest honour graduate. And don't get me started on, 'I was sat!'

MYTH NO. 9. OLD PEOPLE LOOK FOR THINGS TO COMPLAIN ABOUT

Do we really? I guess some people do. Me, for example, in the hairdressers, 'Would you mind turning the music down, it's a bit loud.' 'Sorry? What did you say?' Precisely.

Then there is that old joke about the waiter in a restaurant coming up to a table of elderly ladies and enquiring, 'Is *anything* all right?'

There are certain types of older people who relish passing on bad news and savouring the reaction of the listener. You know the sort of thing: the news is always depressing, the papers are full of stabbings, the weather is terrible, the politicians worse and so on. Their most used phrase is, 'There's always something!' You just want to say, 'Cheer up, it's not so bad!' Fortunately, they are few and far between. Most of the people I know are cheerful and smiley.

However, the universal assumption is that once you reach 50 you are 'invisible', so maybe we object to being seated near the loos in a restaurant out of the way, and being ignored by shop assistants who carry on chatting to each other while we just stand there. I don't really care that men don't whistle at me in the street anymore; if they did – I look quite slim from behind – they would get a big shock when I turned around!

Personally, I quite like being addressed as 'dear' or 'love' by people I don't know such as nurses or checkout staff. I see it simply as a term of informality rather than being patronising. Although it's reported that some older people get sniffy about this, I've never met any who've minded. What *is* irritating is going to the doctor accompanied by my daughter and the doctor discusses my symptoms and treatment with *her* as though I'm senile or invisible!

I promised myself this book would not be a rant against young people and their attitudes: we're all on a continuum from young to old not two separate species, so let's give each other space to be kind.

* * *

Let's look at areas where stereotypes of old people abound: films, television, beauty, fashion and music industries usually portray the elderly as frail, forgetful and always slow. This negative attitude and thinking, including jokes about incontinence and deafness, are generally accepted subjects for humour and nobody turns a hair.

Why are elderly people always seen in magazines, films and commercials with wrinkles, stooped postures and with grey or balding hair? This is reinforced by senior actors being cast as doddery grandparents or grumpy members of society. For example, Grandpa will probably be introduced descending slowly on a stair lift. I guess some progress has been made in the film industry as mature actors are now being cast in more dynamic roles. I was going to mention a couple of them by name but changed my mind in case they died before this book was published!

I suppose it's understandable with a character in a film. The director has a limited time to convey every aspect of a character, therefore, to create an immediate impression of – macho man, scatty woman – stereotypes are used to fill in the details. However, as there are often fewer older characters on screen this often means that stereotypes for older adults are more strongly reinforced.

The over-60s are the largest spending forces in the UK, seeing more films and spending more money, yet they are not represented accordingly. The problem with this is that young people who see these films get a false perception of older people and assume this is how they are and how they should be treated. That is why you often hear someone speaking slowly and in a high-pitched tone to an older person assuming they either have hearing problems or difficulty in understanding what they are saying. This is patronising and disrespectful.

On a larger scale, ageist ideas are often imposed by cultural influences such as media and society in general. For instance, 'anti-ageing' beauty campaigns suggest that everyone should counter ageing and therefore buy products to keep their skin young. Have you notices that these creams and lotions claim to *reduce the appearance* of lines and wrinkles, thereby legally protecting themselves from the fact that they do sod all? As we are bombarded every day with adverts such as this, we are unconsciously being taught to think that young is good and old is bad.

Another dangerous effect of ageing stereotypes is that they can become self-fulfilling prophesies. Our own perceptions of other older people can become self-relevant if we're not careful. If we internalise these negative ageing stereotypes they could influence our cognitive and physical health. This may cause us to restrict our horizons if we see ourselves as 'too old' to pursue certain activities or roles.

Why *are* there so many negative stereotypes? One possibility is fear. Keeping ageing as something to fear creates a market for products such as pills and the cream mentioned above. Fear creates marketing opportunities; seeing 'age' as something to 'put right' is quite an effective strategy.

Surely it is time to fight this and not be sucked in to these beliefs. According to writer Camilla Cavendish in her book *Extra Time*, the Japanese, whose society is now the oldest on the planet, embraced the reality of their elderly citizens years ago. She says that 'Those who are frail and in need of support they call "Old-Old". The group who are still hale and hearty and rushing around after grandchildren they call the "Young-Old", living life to the full in what amounts to an extended middle age. And the two groups need to be treated very differently. We must stop lumping everyone from 60 to 100 together and accept that being vibrant and capable in your 70s is perfectly normal.'

I know which group I'd like to belong to.

Maybe we should also take a leaf out of the book of the good denizens of the Netherlands who have formed a political party called 50PLUS. Its leader MP Henk Krol, born in 1950, stated 'The 50PLUS party was founded by people who thought the elderly had lost their voice in the lower house of the Dutch parliament.' This was set up to campaign for pensioners' rights and so far they have been fighting for the retirement age to be lowered from 66 to 65 (not a battle I would have thought worth the effort), a fixed number of seats for the elderly on public transport (we have that on the tubes which are regularly ignored) and demanding that all trains have lavatories (good one that).

The party is also proposing tax incentives to make it more attractive for young people to have their elderly parents live with them (wouldn't our British Millennials just love that one!) and other policies to persuade companies to train and employ older workers.

I still have a landline – or as I like to call it, a mobile phone finder. I also prefer to pay cash for things rather than use my credit card. I have to confess, though, I do get a smidge impatient when I'm standing behind a youngish person at the ticket machine in an M&S car park clutching my two pound coins and she is paying the same fare with a debit card which takes *forever* to produce the ticket then spews the receipt on to the ground once she's left! It didn't take me long to renege on my promise not to have a rant about young people, did it? Sorry, I must be more careful.

I don't know if you watched that wonderful television series a few years ago called *The Sopranos*? It featured a group of Italian Mafia-type gangsters led by Tony Soprano, played by the sadly deceased James Gandolfini. In a situation say, for example, when they accidentally murdered the wrong person they would give an expansive shrug, assume an expression of mock regret and say, 'So whatcha gonna do?'

Well you are old. So whatcha gonna do? Age is non-negotiable but how you deal with it is up to you. As I say, our culture fosters expectations of an inevitable decline into illness and infirmity. Obviously, you can't reverse ageing chronologically but you can help yourself biologically by concentrating on the age when you felt your most attractive and determine to stay there. It's all in your mind. As the American journalist Andy Rooney said, 'It's paradoxical that the idea of living a long life appeals to everyone but the idea of getting old doesn't appeal to anyone!'

With age comes wisdom, experience, more comfort and security – and the aforementioned travel card. You have increased knowledge about the world and about yourself and a greater understanding of your own resilience. You also have a longer attention span and an increased ability to focus.

Research shows that your sense of what you deem most important for happiness tends to alter appropriately as you age. Priorities shift in a healthy and adaptive fashion, moving away from superficial things and more towards your emotional wellbeing and those you love. You don't really care what other people think, you've developed your own sense of style – or not – and can't believe what idiots are representing us in Parliament. A recent Wellbeing Study of 1,000 men and women aged 70–90 found that in spite of worse physical and cognitive decline, the majority of people felt their wellbeing had improved with age. So, generally, people feel better as they get older.

In this book we will take an irreverent look at what it means to get older and how to improve your life as you go through the years. The anecdotes, experiences and opinions expressed here are largely, but not necessarily, all mine. They are a result of hundreds of conversations with mostly women, rather than men I have to admit, in the 'mature and wise' age group (65–95), as well as experts specialising in geriatric care.

During these conversations it is apparent that one of the main worries and frustrations of people in the above age group is an increased tendency to forget a name. The only reassurance is that everybody seems to be in the same boat. Therefore, I'm sure you will be familiar with the sort of conversation had by three of my companions as we sat round a card table in a local clubhouse playing bridge:

'I was watching that film on Channel Four last night. Did you see it?'

'What was it called?'

'Er, *The Something of Life* – or *The Life of Something* – I can't quite remember.'

'Who was in it?'

'Um, that very good looking guy who was married to that girl from *Friends* and he left her for that woman with six kids, what's her name?'

'Who, Madonna?'

'No, the other one.'

'Madonna was married to Sean Penn.'

'No, it wasn't Sean Penn, this one was younger.'

'I thought Sean Penn was married to Meg Ryan?'

'No that was Tom Hanks.'

'Meg Ryan wasn't in *Friends*.'

'Oh, you know who I mean, he looks a bit like that guy in *Titanic*, um …?'

'Leonardo Di Vinci'

'Yes, but with lighter coloured hair. It'll come to me in a minute…'

'It's not Leonardo Di Vinci – that's the opera singer, you mean Leo di Capricorn.'

'Brad Pitt! That's it!

'That's what?

'In the film.'

'So was it any good?'

'No, it was rubbish.'

And that's what this book is – hopefully not rubbish, but a chat between you and me and my friends which I hope you find amusing and informative. We're all on the same journey, we all have our 'senior moments' but if you can laugh about it, the daily worries and anxieties get pushed to one side for a while. This is your story. You may be old but you don't have to *be* old. As the actress Jane Fonda says: 'I like being over the hill … I've discovered there's a whole new landscape.'

2

THIS WILL HAPPEN TO YOU – BELIEVE IT!

In this chapter we are going to look at what happens to various bodily and mental functions as the years roll by. I have consulted experts in every field of human existence, and I hope you find some of their advice useful.

Please don't shoot the messenger, but I have to report that all your vital organs are going to shrink and/or lose some function as you get older – although it's not as bad as it sounds. Changes do occur in the body's cells, tissues and organs, and those changes can affect functioning of all body systems to some degree, from your eyes and ears to diminishing taste buds and sense of smell. This is natural and normal and happens to everyone. Where once you would strive for improvement, in the end it becomes a quest for maintenance.

So whatcha gonna do?!

YOUR BRAIN AND YOUR MEMORY

There is a cartoon on my wall depicting a group of older women waving placards and chanting in a protest march. There are four squares:

Square 1. 'WHAT DO WE WANT?'
Square 2. 'A BETTER MEMORY!'
Square 3. 'WHEN DO WE WANT IT?'
Square 4. 'WANT WHAT?'

Let me ask you: Do you have a large hippocampus? Answer: you may have done once but now, well, you're not so sure! Your hippocampus is part of the limbic system in your brain which is responsible for processing and storage of short and long-term memory. It is also the region that regulates emotions, which is why events which would have thrown you into a right old tizzy when you were younger are now viewed with a stoic shrug.

You also have another memory storage facility in your brain: the prefrontal cortex. This records the same event as the hippocampus while it's happening, but it takes longer to process it, maybe taking up to two weeks to fully imprint the details in your cortex. During this time, the memory of the same event in the hippocampus fades slightly. This means you have two slightly different memories of what happened in your mind.

Scientists believe that as you get older, there is a shift in the balance of the two memory storage systems. Therefore, should someone ask you about a particular event, you may recount one of two different versions depending on which area of the brain is engaged at the time – which may explain why your memory can get a bit fuzzy sometimes.

Let's talk a bit more about that elusive memory. I'm sure you're not as ditsy as my friends were pretending (?) to be in the last chapter, but I know how scary it is when you are having a normal conversation with someone and suddenly the word you are searching for to describe something totally eludes you. It's an ordinary everyday word you have used a thousand times – what was it? You experience a slight flash of panic which makes things worse as you are now focusing on the panicky feeling rather than the word you are trying to remember. A few minutes later, once you have calmed down, it pops back into your mind again. Please don't worry, this happens to everyone.

Another strange occurrence is when you mean to say one thing and another word, quite similar to the one you meant to use, comes out instead. Whoa! What's that about? Are you going mad, is this the first sign of dementia? And don't even mention remembering people's names ten seconds after you have been introduced!

Well, you are not going mad, nor are you getting Alzheimer's. According to clinical neuropsychologist Ylva Ostby who, with her novelist sister, Hilde, has written a book with the catchy title, *Adventures in Memory, the Science of Remembering and Forgetting*, (I bet you won't remember that!) a certain amount of forgetfulness is essential for a healthy brain. She states that forgetting certain types of information is the brain's way of protecting itself from overload. However, that's not much help when you are introducing your cousin Helen to your husband and her name has vanished from your memory – or, even worse, *his*!

Your brain actually starts ageing in your 20s, steadily losing the neurons, which are the cells which make up the brain and nervous system. Don't worry though, you have millions of them, and although by your 60s your brain has shrunk somewhat, you are still a perfectly normal functioning human being, fully in control of all your faculties.

Modern life, including the internet, television, 24-hour news channels and mobile phones means that we are exposed to a barrage of information throughout the day. Not only is it normal for our brain to discard most of it, it's also desirable. If it didn't, our system would be overloaded, and your brain would probably explode (not a scientific fact!)

As for remembering names it all depends on how important that person is to you. Your memory keeps hold of information for only a few seconds, or for as long as you keep thinking of it. The book states that when you meet someone you are filling up your memory with a lot of other information such as how you might appear to them, what you are going to say next and what it would be like to have sex with them (I made that last one up). The way to overcome this is to repeat their name as soon as you hear it: 'How nice to meet you Peter', 'Do you live round here Peter?' and try and associate a physical attachment to the name: 'Peter dandruff' for example. Though the next time you meet him you might say, 'Hello Dan.'

This sort of problem affects both men and women equally, although men are also prone to suffer from something known as 'male pattern blindness.' For example, my husband would stand in front of the open fridge gazing inside, then say, 'Where's the cheese?' I'd reply 'Right there in front of you.' He just can't see it. Why? Because it happens to be on a different shelf in the fridge that day. My fault. I wonder if there is a scientific study somewhere that proves women blame themselves for everything that happens whereas men look for blame elsewhere. For example, I would say 'I can't find my glasses' whereas he would say, 'What have you done with my glasses?' My fault. They say behind every successful man is a woman – and behind her is his wife!

Lost keys are a common occurrence in every household. You *know* you put them down on the hall table but they're nowhere to be found, and you get more irritated by the minute as you search from room to room. Putting keys down is a mundane activity, which doesn't require concentration. Your brain simply isn't paying attention to it. If you're not aware of what you are doing, the information can't enter your long-term memory.

I know it's stating the obvious but put your keys in the same place *every time* you come home, preferably in a rather quirky place, but where you can see them, such as an empty jam jar in the place where you hang your coat.

You can also help yourself by saying an action out loud. When I take something out of the oven, I say 'off' as I turn the knob. This saves me coming down in the middle of the night to check. The same advice is relevant when you park your car. Saying out loud 'By the third pillar on the right, near the blue door' will stop you wandering round the car park pointing your keys at similar makes hoping one will 'bleep.'

When leaving your house, just before you shut the front door behind you, say 'bag', 'phone' and 'keys' to make sure you have these with you. I know I'm suggesting you sound like a raving nutter talking to yourself, but at least you won't lock yourself out.

We all have too much to do and think about today which makes it difficult for the brain to filter what is important to retain and what needs to be taken out. Younger people keep all appointments on their mobile phones as an external memory aid. I can't do that. I have to have everything written down either in a desk diary that I check every day, or a large notebook where I jot down things I need to do, people I have to call. By writing something down it is attaching meaning to this specific piece of information, so you can then 'tick it off', both literally and in your head. Even then, your mind is so full of things you have to do that most people go through the day on automatic pilot without fully concentrating on what they're doing and hope for the best.

The danger of this is aptly illustrated by the recent experience of my friend, Nancy (not her real name ... actually, it is!). She was visiting her local shopping centre and chose a lovely dress in Zara. There was such a queue for the changing room that she bought it in two sizes to try on at home. Having chosen the one that fitted best she went back the next day to return the other one. Before she did that, she bought a wedding present for a friend's daughter in Fenwick which was on an upper floor.

Finally reaching the front of the queue at Zara, Nancy discovered she had left her credit card in the machine in Fenwick. She panicked and ran up the escalator to the store. Luckily her card was still in the machine, (phew!) and by the time she had lectured the poor assistant as to why they don't hand you back your credit card with your receipt as other stores do rather than relying on you to remove it yourself, she realised she had left the wedding present in a huge bag in the queue at Zara! Back down the escalator she raced and there was the bag, plonked on the floor where she had left it. Fortunately no one had spotted it. She had to buy a Krispy Kreme doughnut to calm herself down.

TRAIN YOUR BRAIN

You've read about the necessity of keeping your brain actively engaged if you want to enhance your memory so would you say doing crossword puzzles and Sudoku are beneficial for your brain or not? Will it stop you going doo-lally? One minute we're told that learning a new language is the key for preventing dementia, the next minute we're told that the brain is not a muscle and you can't 'train' it by completing the *Times* crossword every day.

Cognitive neuroscientist, Dr Sabina Brennan, in her book *100 Days to a Younger Brain* suggests that while some training produces statistically significant improvement in the practised skill, claims made for promoting brain games are frequently exaggerated and at times misleading. She prefers advising people to concentrate on social activities and learning new skills rather than playing Sudoku. (Surely you can do both?)

Conversely, most scientists suggest that doing puzzles *does* work – at least partly. Scientists at Aberdeen University conducted a series of cognitive studies which were published in the 2018 Christmas edition of the *British Medical Journal*. They state that regularly engaging in intellectual activities boosts mental ability throughout life and provides a 'higher cognitive point' from which to decline. Although this won't stop you getting dementia eventually if it's on the cards, it does raise the point at which dementia-type symptoms start, meaning that an individual stays mentally astute for longer. That's good news.

What they are saying is that the brain has great plasticity; it is constantly growing, changing and adapting throughout our lives. Regardless of what age you are, your brain will retain this capacity, although it does slow down and more nerve connections are lost than created. However, it's not the number of brain cells – neurons – you have but the strength of the connections between those cells that determine your thinking power, or cognitive function.

This study shows that regularly using the brain for complex tasks – including practising memory games and other mental challenges – both creates and strengthens a greater number of connections between the brain cells. It does this by releasing proteins called neurotrophic growth factors which help neurons survive and reproduce. Even small challenges like cleaning your teeth by holding the toothbrush in the other hand can achieve the same result by focusing your mind on what you're doing (are you listening, Nancy?). All these activities stimulate cumulative memories in your brain making it more efficient in remembering important things.

Evidence suggests that the best brain boosting activities are creative, especially those which involve visual and motor skills – that is, using your hands for painting, sculpting, basket weaving etc. Therefore, if, heaven forbid, you do get dementia, you have a backup of neurons in your brain to slow down the development.

My friend Celia loves getting her hands into wet clay at her pottery classes and we've all been presented with a series of wonky pots which seem to be the sole attainment of her artistic ability. Another friend, Mims, is hooked on cross stitch embroidery. She's gone past kittens and flowers and now presents her friends with cushion covers sporting some choice swear words and their definitions.

It's worth persevering at any chosen activity. Although I have been teaching myself to play the piano for some time now, I am still total rubbish at it but it keeps my mind focused and I love bashing out my own version of blues and jazz. I do use headphones though, out of respect for my neighbours.

One of the most important things you can do for the health of your brain and your body is *exercise* which not only keeps you fit but may fend off many diseases that older people suffer from, including signs of ageing. We will come to that in more detail in a later chapter.

DEAL WITH WORRY

With every year that goes by your worry quota increases exponentially. Every day the newspapers seem to report yet another senseless stabbing of an innocent person in the street or children being blown up in an arena listening to their favourite singer.

Every atrocity sears itself into your mind as you think of your beloved grandchildren growing up in this violent world and you worry about them endlessly, especially when you can't sleep. You imagine terrible things happening to them which go round and round in a continuous loop in your mind until your whole being is fraught with tension.

Don't let this become overwhelming to the point it can impact on your enjoyment of life. These are thoughts not predictions and chances are they won't happen.

If by worrying you could prevent some catastrophe from happening, it might be worthwhile. But worry is a destructive emotion and the only person it negatively affects is you – and it shows on your face.

Deal with it: Confront your 'what if' situations in a calm, rational manner. For example, your 17-year-old granddaughter is planning a gap year travelling to far-flung countries before taking up her place at university. Your mind plays terrible tricks recalling pictures of grieving parents flying to collect their child's body from some godforsaken place and won't let the image go.

STOP. First, bring your mind back to the here and now. Ask yourself: where is your granddaughter at this minute? Probably at home in her bedroom excitedly Instagramming pictures of her *amazing* new haircut by this cool new guy she's discovered who is so, like, *buff*, you know, with *amazing* hair (see selfie) and she can't wait for all her 600 friends to reply telling her that she looks *a-ma-zing*!

Next – reality check. Remind yourself that thousands of young people go travelling every year and come back safe and sound. They either go with a friend or meet up with similar young people along the way and they all stick together and watch out and protect each other. Also, with today's technology, everyone can be contacted at the touch of a button.

Do you get it? Take your 'what ifs' to their logical conclusions and banish them from your mind. I know it's not always easy but if this advice helps to alleviate your fears, I'm glad.

That's it with the mental changes that accumulate and accelerate with age. Let's have a look at some of the physical changes that you may have noticed as the years creep by, such as:

YOUR FACE/SKIN

In your 20s you just didn't appreciate your collagen-rich smooth skin and the subcutaneous fat below the surface which shaped your lovely face. This precious commodity slowly decreases so by the time you are 40, you have lost a bit of volume in your face and drier skin makes the fine lines around your eyes more visible.

In my case, by the time I hit 50 it felt like my face was 'falling off' and gathering under my chin! So I did something about it. I'm not suggesting you follow my example and have a facelift, but it did make me feel so much better, although now I'm in my 80s there is a definite softening of my jawline. I certainly wouldn't do anything further about it now; have you seen the horrors on your TV screen every day! What's with the gigantic pouty lips?!

I have not experimented with Botox either as I am reluctant to introduce a paralysing agent into my body. I realise that Botox is injected into a specific muscle group for the sole purpose of preventing those muscles from excessive movement, thereby eliminating frown lines and wrinkles round your eyes when you smile.

The actual drug has been used for many years and is extremely beneficial for those people affected by an involuntary movement, such as a tic in the face. I know that only minuscule amounts are used, and presumably the drug stays *in situ*, thereby making a mockery of my fanciful notion that anything injected into the body must get into the bloodstream and therefore circulate to other organs including the brain. With my family history of dementia, the last thing I want is for my brain to become paralysed!

May I state categorically this is *not* a proven or medical fact – only my own, probably totally inaccurate conjecture – so if you want to try Botox please don't let me dissuade you. For me, it is always obvious when someone is a regular user by their shiny, slightly bulgy forehead and the 'bunny lines' at the sides of their nose when they laugh. After all, the wrinkles have to go somewhere!

Other non-invasive treatments, such as fillers like Restylane, are placed just under the skin to smooth out lines and wrinkles and these generally give good – albeit temporary – results, although the area can look a little lumpy in the hands of an unqualified practitioner. Which is why, if you are going to have anything done to your face, non-invasive or otherwise, please, I implore you, do go to a reputable plastic surgeon even if it is more expensive than your local salon, and even if said salon employs a 'qualified nurse' to wield the syringe. Do not take risks with your face – it's the face your family love.

As a lesser option, my friends and I have tried all the creams and anti-ageing potions but nothing really works in the long term; anything that could penetrate the skin deeper than the surface level would be classified as a drug and need a prescription.

You know that smoking causes wrinkles, especially those little vertical lines around your mouth from constantly pursing your lips. Obviously if you're going to lie out in the sun for hours, you're asking for trouble; the word 'tanning' means to thicken and harden. But we all know women who think that sundried all-the-year-round tan is attractive – or is it just their way of telling you they either own homes abroad or decamp to further sunny shores during the British dismal winter? Who can blame them! Personally, I don't think it's worth that crepey chest.

I do know that a diet containing a lot of refined sugar can hasten the glycation process and make your skin look sallow and older. Glycation happens when the refined sugar found in cakes, biscuits, chocolate – just think of everything you like – reacts with proteins and fats in an abnormal way, producing harmful molecules called 'advanced glycation end-products' (conveniently and appropriately known by the acronym: AGEs). The more AGEs you have in your body, the more it affects production of collagen, which gives skin its firmness, and elastin, which helps skin bounce back after being stretched.

The *British Journal of Dermatology* reports that after the age of 35, glycation in the skin increases and continues to do so as you get older. Worse, when your skin is exposed to UV rays, it accelerates glycation, further ageing the skin and causing those brown age spots and uneven skin tones.

You know the answer! To keep your skin looking younger for longer, cut down on foods containing refined sugar, drink plenty of water to keep your skin hydrated and when you do go out in the sun, slather on the sunscreen, always wear a hat and cover up as much as possible. Sorry to be such a spoilsport but it's your choice.

Much as I'm keen on exercise, I don't advise doing facial exercises advocated by the occasional female celebrity popping up in a magazine or newspaper, claiming it's that which is making her look so much younger than her age – rather than the more truthful airbrushing. Your facial muscles are attached to your skin whereas the other muscles in your body are fixed to your bones with tendons. You can't 'tone' your facial muscles in this way and screwing up your face will only add more lines. You are using your facial muscles all the time with every expression you make as well as when you eat – and nobody I know has bulgy facial muscles! You?

I guess it's just a matter of having good genes whether you inherit very dry skin which wrinkles easily, or smoother skin which takes a little longer to dry out. Just be kind to your face – it's the only one you have.

FACIAL HAIR

Has this happened to you? You are rinsing your face with water and your hand brushes against something small on your lower jaw. What is it, a spot? You dry your face and look more closely in the magnifying mirror. Good Lord, it's a hard little bristle! Coming out of your *face*! What the…? Is this normal? Are you growing a beard? Do you need to join the circus?

OK, calm down. Welcome to yet another manifestation of the myriad changes as you get older. As the hair on your head gets thinner, it compensates by sprouting in other places. I believe it was Joan Rivers who said she brushed a hair off her shoulder and found it was still attached to her chin.

You grab some tweezers and remove it and forget about it – until it happens again, and again and, for some unfortunate women, it becomes a veritable forest. However, help is at hand and you can easily have the area of your chin and moustache threaded or waxed for as little as ten pounds. Or for a similar price you can invest in a marvellous little implement called a Kapmore Effective Epilator kit which is a thick spring coil with handles at either end. You trap the hair in the coil and rip it out by the root. Lots of fun to be had there.

There are more permanent solutions such as laser hair removal, which used to be only effective if the hair is dark, but they might have changed the technology now, and electrolysis.

The only compensation is that at least the hairs on your legs and under your arms get sparser, although the length remains the same, and you won't need a bikini wax – unless there's something you're not telling me?

YOUR TEETH

Your teeth are actually very strong. When you consider all the biting, chewing and grinding you do, it's surprising the enamel doesn't wear out much quicker than it does. Your gums do gradually recede with age though, which inspires the description of an old person as being 'long in the tooth.' This means you are at greater risk of tooth decay near the roots as food can get stuck in the little gaps in this area.

When I've finished a meal in a restaurant, I think to myself 'That was nice; I'll take the rest of it home in my teeth for later.' I'm sure you, like me, can't wait to get home to find a toothpick to remove the debris; this is something you would never do in public however surreptitiously.

British people are famed – and mocked – for their 'yellow' teeth which are partly a result of loss of surface enamel and staining from tea, coffee and foods containing substances like turmeric we eat on a regular basis. Citrus fruits and carbonated drinks dissolve this protective enamel making dental cavities more prevalent near the gum line.

Teeth whitening salons are opening up all over the country. In the UK, only dental professionals registered with the General Dental Council (GDC) can legally carry out teeth whitening. There are two methods available, the more expensive one performed in a clinic involves a solution of hydrogen peroxide and either a laser or LED. Results are immediate and prices in London range from £600 to £1,000. The second requires specially moulded trays and a similar, albeit weaker, formula that can be dispensed and administered at home. This takes longer for results to become apparent – approximately two weeks – and costs around £300. Some of these 'at home' kits can be ordered online which can pose serious risks to the consumer as many contain far higher percentages of hydrogen peroxide which can really damage the teeth. Also, any hairdresser or beautician performing teeth whitening is likely doing so illegally with the courts handing out increasingly severe fines for convictions.

Most of my friends have asked their dentists if they can lighten their teeth just a bit, not the glaring white which would look odd, but just to make them look a brighter version of the colour they have. A reputable dentist will advise against messing about with the colour as this procedure can be detrimental to older people. As the gums shrink, more of the soft root tissue at the neck of the tooth is exposed. This could make tooth whitening extremely painful and the bleaching chemicals used in this process could cause permanent sensitivity and even damage the teeth irrevocably. I'd rather my teeth were in my mouth than in the bin whatever the colour. Personally, I think those gleaming white teeth sported by certain television personalities look more false than actual false teeth, don't you?

The worst things for your teeth are, as you know, foods containing refined sugar and fruit drinks. But did you know that as you get older you produce less moisture in your mouth and this can also contribute to cavities forming? Dry mouth is also caused by certain medications including those for asthma, high blood pressure and cholesterol or Parkinson's disease. That is why your dentist always enquires if you are taking any medication and it's why you are advised to drink plenty of water to keep your mouth lubricated.

Hopefully most people do have a dental check every six months and maybe a separate visit to a dental hygienist to get their teeth thoroughly cleaned. As my old dentist once said to me, 'when you lose your teeth, the sun goes out.' I'm not quite sure how losing your teeth can affect the solar system but I knew what he meant: you should hang on to your homegrown teeth as long as possible because dentures are a pain.

To this end I'm sure, like me, you have an array of flossing tape and little interdental brushes of all sizes. When I was younger it took me three minutes to clean my teeth and get into bed; now it takes ten minutes and it's such a drag.

If you do have to have a tooth extracted, please consider a dental implant. This is a titanium screw – with a visible tooth crown – fixed into the jawbone. I know they are hideously expensive but if you can afford it and your jawbone is strong enough, do enquire about it with your dentist. The result is a proper tooth where there was once a gap, which feels so natural you forget that you haven't grown it yourself. As the bone and gum grow round the implant, this keeps that area healthy. If you leave the gap, the gum may eventually shrink causing the tooth next to it to become wobbly and your cheeks start to get that hollow look making you appear even older. Just saying...

YOUR ARMS

The arms! Oh dear, the arms – the part of the body older women moan about the most. You'll know what I mean when you stand at your front door waving goodbye to your grandchildren and your upper arm continues waving even when they have turned the corner.

Sadly, at some point in your 60s or 70s your arms will 'go.' The skin on your upper arms will change from being smooth and unblemished to lined and wrinkled and the flesh underneath becomes soft, seemingly overnight. It's as though your arms suddenly belong to someone else, someone aged about 100 who bears no relation to how you see yourself. This happens to all women, both fat and slim and there is nothing you can do about it. You either flaunt it or hide it.

The doyenne of fashion, Anna Wintour, has obviously decided 'to hell with it' and continues to wear sleeveless dresses in her 70s with the confidence of knowing no one would dare mention anything about it. Good for her.

The only thing you can do is to keep the muscles in your arms toned so ensuring a good shape which does lessen the effect of the overlying skin. I'll tell you which exercises work for that in more detail in a later chapter. Creams and anti-cellulite lotions don't work, plastic surgery is possible but, as with any surgery, it will leave a huge scar, although mostly hidden in your armpit. I wouldn't go there.

Women complain about the same thing happening on their inner thighs – I've heard them likened to porridge – but at least these aren't on show the whole time. Well, maybe yours are – I don't want to know.

YOUR BLADDER

Suddenly your bladder develops a mind of its own. You can be out shopping, or doing whatever for a whole morning without needing the loo but the *moment* you step into the house you need to go – urgently – like *now*. Sometimes you just drop your coat and keys on the floor to get there in time. What's that about?

It's the reduction of oestrogen after the menopause which causes the scary-sounding 'urinary atrophy incontinence.' This is medico-speak for when you cough or sneeze violently you sometimes get a 'wet penny.' Definition: a little blot of escaped urine which will irritate you so much you feel compelled to change into a fresh pair of knicks then and there. Bit embarrassing in Costa.

Another thing my friends and I have noticed, apart from infections like interstitial cystitis, thrush and bacterial vaginosis (isn't it fun being a woman!) is that the messages from the brain dictating your toilet needs are much weaker. You know when you need to go, but what you're not sure about is when you have finished and it's safe to stand up! Has this happened to you?

Sorry to be so graphic but you're sitting on the loo after a satisfactory flow and think you're done. So you stand up and start doing the necessary to get yourself in order, but suddenly realise the bladder hasn't finished emptying itself and you have to reverse what you're doing and sit back down. So annoying.

The solution decreed by my group of friends is: you sit there a bit longer and sing 'Happy Birthday' all the way through twice, and if nothing happens after that, it's safe to stand up and pull up. You're welcome.

YOUR BREASTS

You would think that the face is the part that ages fastest, but in fact, it is your breasts which are the most sensitive to the ageing process. They get bigger when you put on weight or get pregnant and lose density as you lose weight or breastfeed and the skin reacts accordingly.

I'm not going into the merits – or otherwise – of breast implants, except to say that breast cancer is more prevalent in a woman's later years and implants may impede detection of tumours during a mammogram or scan. After a mastectomy you would obviously be guided by your surgeon as to whether implants or surgical reconstruction is advisable.

My friend Dilly and I were having a conversation as to whether it is permissible to go braless at our age when wearing a low-cut dress or top. I have always extolled the merits of wearing a soft bra in bed which I have done since becoming pregnant with my first child at age 19. I just find it more comfortable than flopping around every time I turn over, and my breasts, although smaller, are still roughly in the same place on my chest they always were. Dilly claims this is unnecessary as your breasts don't flop around that much in bed and anyway, her husband likes to ... I don't want to know!

We decided to do the pencil test to settle the argument – you know the one: you put a pencil under your naked breast and if it falls down (the pencil that is) then you're perky enough to go braless. If it stays where it is, you're too saggy. My pencil fell straight to the floor. Dilly is still looking for hers!

YOUR BONES

It's that stupid menopause again which strips your bones of the minerals that gave you the strength to run around the tennis court and stomp up and down hills without your legs aching. Your bones might feel solid, but the inside of the bone is like honeycomb. This is not static as bone tissue is being built up and broken down all the time.

Problems arise when we break down more bone than we build up and the tiny holes within the bones get bigger until they resemble Swiss cheese. The solid outer layer gets thinner as well so your bones get less dense. If this goes too far then you're into osteoporosis territory. I think bone density scans for the hip and spine should be available for everyone over 65 but the NHS appear to want to wait until you break something before you can have one to determine whether you are a candidate for the bisphosphonate drugs that fight bone loss.

You may have noticed that whenever your grandchildren visit, they seem to have grown taller. Possibly they have but it's also you who have become shorter. Both men and women lose height as they get older: between the ages of 50–70 men lose approximately one inch and women lose two inches. This is because it's not only the bones in your arms and legs that get more porous as you get older. The vertebrae comprising your spine and skeletal system also loses minerals and the discs between the vertebrae get thinner causing the chunks of bone to become compressed. This accounts for the 'little old lady' tag which, when you think about it, is fairly accurate as there are few very tall old people.

Although less solid, the long bones in your arms and legs stay the same length so, as your trunk gets shorter, your arms appear longer, therefore by the time you reach 100 you could be walking with your knuckles scraping the floor! Sadly, changes in the joints affect almost all old people, ranging from minor stiffness to severe arthritis which can be seen in the thickening joints in fingers and knuckles.

For most elderly people, the bones should be strong enough to withstand a fall without breaking. If they are weak, it all depends on the way you fall. Wrist fractures happen when you fall forwards or backwards and put your hands out to break the fall. Hip fractures happen when you fall sideways. So, if you insist on leaving that wire from the electric fire or fan trailing in the doorway, you can choose which bit you want to break.

The best way to prevent all this happening is *exercise*! We'll come to that...

YOUR FINGER AND TOENAILS

What has happened to your toenails?! From a quick snip round with the scissors, it now takes an industrial strength tool to hack through them. Toenails get thicker because of the accumulation of nail cells called onychocytes. As Michael Caine didn't say: 'not a lot of people know that.'

You may be prone to get fungal infections on your toenails, which are very common as fungus thrives in the dark moist environment inside shoes, and there is not much you can do about that.

Fingernails don't thicken like toenails, fortunately, but they do get dry causing ridges of vertical lines to develop, which split and catch on your clothes which is very annoying. All you can do is keep your nails lubricated and soft by rubbing in cuticle oil containing vitamin E and use a heavy hand cream. The supplement biotin helps keep hair, skin and nails healthy. The other option, adopted by many fashion-conscious women is to have false nails – sorry, 'artificial nail enhancements' – stuck on to their own fingertips. These can be made from acrylic plastic or the more natural-looking gel nails. Neither of these actually harm the nail bed although in older people they can cause the actual nails to become thin, brittle and dry. Dermatologists advise choosing the soak off gel nails which are kinder to the actual nails then the acrylic plastic ones which, apparently, are a bugger to remove.

YOUR STOMACH SHAPE

How many women over 60 do you see who look about seven months pregnant? I've seen plenty, including my friend Dilly, whose tummy arrives at her destination a few seconds before she does. As she says, 'I'm fat but I identify as skinny, so I guess that makes me trans-fat.' She's funny, my friend Dilly.

It's the fault of that menopause again, causing decreased levels of oestrogen which influence where fat is distributed in the body. Less oestrogen means the small amount of the male hormone, testosterone, that women have, comes to the fore and the body develops a more masculine fat tummy shape. The problem is not limited to the extra layer of blubber just below the skin – subcutaneous fat – but also includes visceral fat lying deep in the abdomen surrounding the internal organs. This is both unattractive and unhealthy and can leave you more prone to developing heart disease, diabetes and other health problems. All the women I have spoken to find men with huge stomachs protruding above a belt, trying vainly to hold up their trousers, grossly revolting and we all wonder how they can find their ... never mind. With women, who often have slim legs below the bulge, the necessity of wearing a voluminous top gives the whole shape the appearance of a barrel on legs.

Do this: sling a tape measure round what was once your waist. If the measurement is over 35 inches (89 centimetres) it indicates an unhealthy concentration of fat in this area and you need to think about losing weight, girl! If the tape measure is too short to go all the way round, you are definitely in trouble. However, visceral fat responds to the same diet and exercise strategies that help you lower total body fat.

YOUR GENERAL HEALTH

For some reason the National Health Service stops summoning you for regular breast screening once you reach 70. This is a bit short-sighted as most breast cancers appear after that age. For this reason, my advice is to take charge of it yourself. I have a mammogram and a gynaecological check every three years and pay to have this done privately. I have lost too many lovely friends to cancer to take risks with my health. I have the greatest respect for the NHS and admiration for everyone who works for it; doctors at my local hospital saved my husband's life on more than one occasion. Your own GP will refer you to get these checks done under the NHS but only if you have symptoms, and then it takes so long to see a consultant that something that should have been diagnosed months ago could have spread. I would rather spend less money on other things and keep up my private health insurance.

Even if you have had a hysterectomy it is still worth having a gynae check every few years. I had a hysterectomy at age 50 and that, and the facelift, were the best things I have ever done under an anaesthetic! After having five children my womb was practically dropping out on the floor, so I was able to have a vaginal hysterectomy without the need for an incision. This meant a far quicker recovery and I was able to leave hospital after three days and was back teaching my exercise class after three weeks.

However, that means I still have ovaries, so I submit myself for a scan every three years and advise you to do the same, whether privately or on the NHS. I know it's unpleasant lying there as the practitioner puts a condom on to a suitably shaped gadget and sticks it up you-know-where, but this detects any dodgy lumps and bumps in your inside and measures any small ovarian cysts that may become troublesome in later years. Even without a womb you still need to have a smear test and provide a urine sample to check for diabetes.

Please don't dismiss any symptoms, be they a funny looking mark on your skin, a persistent cough, pain, or occasional suspicious bleeding from any orifice. I know it's a drag to contemplate the arduous process of trying to get an appointment with your GP, and although I hate the anachronisms young people use in texting, FOFO – Fear of Finding Out – is a psychological trait to which we Brits are horribly susceptible. This explains why a review of the past twenty years of cancer care by the Health Foundation charity found that the survival rate in the UK lags behind many other countries.

There is no point in my telling you not to Google your symptoms because I know you will. Lots of women my age suffer from Googleitis Neurosa. This is where you get a twinge in your calf and look up your symptoms online. By the time you have browsed several medical websites you are convinced you not only have deep vein thrombosis but have only hours to live. The answer is to visit your doctor and sit there while he/she looks up your symptoms on Google. Seriously, don't self-diagnose because you may either gain false reassurance by doing this, or be needlessly scared. Let the doc sort it out and don't be put off if their attitude is dismissive and you still feel uneasy. Many older people can be rather too timid and respectful towards the medical profession to question their diagnosis as they 'don't want to be a bother.' Well, be a bother, girl! I know that if you, like me, were brought up as a good 50s house-wife, it is in your nature to be compliant and not speak up for your rights. Well, as far as your health is concerned, sod that! This is especially important if you need an oper-ation and you sense the doctors hesitating because of your age. An elderly aunt of mine suffered from diverticulosis for years and had to enlist her GP grandson to speak up on her behalf when the doctors were not forthcoming with an operation. She had it and lived to 101.

SEX

When I mentioned to friends I was writing a book about older people and health, several said 'Oh you have to include a section about sex.' No. I don't. I've always considered intercourse to be a loving and private act between two people. It's none of my business, nor yours. None of us can comprehend how the modern generation have such a casual attitude towards sex – just something to do if you're bored, or the natural end to an evening even if you have just met that person a few hours ago.

I deplore that sex has become so explicit on TV and cinema screens with each (probably male) director trying to increase the shock quota. Talking of that, is it only in TV dramas that a couple start getting amorous in the kitchen and the man hoists the woman up on a table or the work surface amongst the dirty crockery and proceeds to have sex with her like that? I may be totally naïve about the swinging from the chandelier type of sexual experience, but I do have a pretty good idea of what goes where! So how do they manage it in that position? Just a thought.

I do get irritated by glamorous older stars declaring they are 'having the best sex of their lives' with their latest toy boy. No, they're not – unless their vaginas have developed their own internal lubricating system that has bypassed the rest of us. At least Jane Fonda (her real name) had the decency, once she hit 80, to say 'That's it, I've shut up shop down there.' I wish the rest of them would just shut up. Having said that, I've been proved wrong by reading that the NHS is launching a campaign for free condoms to be handed out to pensioners at GP surgeries and community centres to cut down the escalating spread of sexually transmitted diseases amongst old people. What?!This is on the advice of the International Longevity Centre UK, which has reported that women, in particular, find it easier to become aroused in their 80s than in their 60s and 70s. How do they know? Are we supposed to believe there are thousands of elderly people furiously at it like rabbits with multiple partners? As mentioned above, I've obviously led a sheltered life. At my age, 'getting lucky' is walking into a room and remembering what I came in for!

Wait, there's more: guidelines published by the Royal College of Nursing in 2018 suggest that care homes – *care homes!* – should put aside private rooms for elderly residents in their 90s to have sex, complete with double beds and 'do not disturb signs.' Oh, leave it out! My Auntie Sonia, who suffered from advanced Alzheimer's, was in a care home until she died, aged 93 last year and I cannot for the life of me imagine any of the other randy resident Lotharios knocking on her door for a quickie. They would have to remove their catheters first!

I discussed this with my friend Joan whose 93-year-old father is currently in a care home. A former doctor, he is mentally confused rather than having full-blown Alzheimer's and couldn't manage on his own after Joan's mother died. He has become attracted to a lady of similar age in the home and is convinced that she is his wife. The lady herself doesn't appear to contest this and they sit together in the day room holding hands, which is rather sweet. The staff told Joan that they cuddle up together on his bed for an afternoon nap although they are separated at night. The problem is that when Joan and her family take her dad out for lunch, which they do every Sunday, he insists that they take this lady along with them, and as she has a hearty appetite it rather bumps up the bill at the end of the meal! As long as her dad is happy though, they don't mind.

YOUR EYES AND EARS

As you have probably observed, your eyes are the first thing that need attention as your vision changes as early as 40. The usual symptoms are trouble seeing closeup, reading, threading needles etc. Obviously, an eye test reveals whether you need glasses or not and most people do, either for short or long-sightedness. During your eye test you will also be checked for dry eyes, glaucoma, cataracts and macular degeneration and given the information you need to deal with any problems that arise. That's why it's so important not to ignore those yearly reminders.

'Grandma, you've got such big ears', is a common observation from a vocally filter-free grandchild – and they're right. Your ears keep on growing throughout your life, more in length than width, and men's ears grow more than women's. Your bones stop growing once you reach puberty, but cartilage – which your ears are made of – continues to grow, slowly, until you die. Gravity also plays a part, as does wearing heavy dangly earrings. Fortunately, not many people are as observant as small children and don't notice this phenomenon.

They might also mention your nose which, although it doesn't get bigger, it just looks as if it does because your face gets thinner. You might need to keep a tissue handy for the drip that occasionally appears on the tip of your nose (why?) – such a nuisance.

As for your hearing, in my opinion people speak too softly in company and shout too loudly in restaurants. Cinema adverts and trailers are deafening: 'EXPERIENCE DOLBY SOUND: BOOM! BOOM! BOOM!' – the floor actually vibrates! Do they think this adds to the enjoyment of your visit? Likewise, with strobing lights flashing into your eyes – who are the morons that think this is pleasurable? Are they on drugs?

If you haven't decided to throw yourself under a bus after reading this chapter, I'll tell you what happened to me when I had started having problems with my hearing.

3

ARE YOU DEAF OR WHAT?

It started with my daughter saying to me: 'Widdy you neater lev viz slough, weave gotta sutt tie ton?'

I said, 'What did you say?'

She sighed. 'I SAID, WHY DO YOU NEED THE TELEVISION SO LOUD WHEN YOU'VE GOT THE SUBTITLES ON?'

I gestured towards the screen. 'Because I can't make out what she's saying. She's just mumbling.'

To which my daughter replied, 'How can she be mumbling – she's the Queen!'

Thinking about it later I did sometimes strain to hear what people were saying, especially when they drop their voices at the end of a sentence. And admittedly, I do have the television quite loud, but I thought it was their fault for not getting the sound quality right.

I decided to take advantage of the offer of a free hearing test at Boots at my local shopping centre where I get my glasses. The Optical and Hearing Aid Centre is situated at the back of the store where there is a little hallway and a staircase leading up to a large area, with three walls covered with increasingly expensive spectacle frames.

I approached the counter and stood behind a lady also waiting for attention. Eventually a young man stopped pretending to be busy and said, 'Can I help you?' The lady said 'Yes, I've come for my hearing test.' The young man looked in the appointment book and said, 'Right, what's your name?' She said 'Pardon?'

I gave a snort of laughter which I hastily turned into a cough, obviously unsuccessfully as she glared at me. I made an appointment for the following week and sent a text to my daughter, 'You'll be pleased to know I'm getting some hearing aids.' She texted back 'That should keep you warm.' I thought, what is she talking about? I checked my wording and found I had informed her I was getting some 'heating aids.' Stupid phone!

It was raining the day of my appointment and I must have looked a bit bedraggled as I walked through the store towards the back, only to be confronted by a group of Boots executives – about seven or eight smartly dressed men and women standing in the hallway having a chat. I hesitated and one of the men stepped back politely indicating I should go up the stairs. But I'm afraid my inner stand-up comedian took over my brain at that point and I looked round at their serious faces and announced: 'Right, well, I expect you're all wondering why I've called this meeting.' There was a split second of startled silence as they regarded this clearly deranged woman standing there clutching a dripping umbrella, then, as one, they exploded into gales of prolonged laughter – probably because it was so unexpected – but I could still hear them laughing as I went up the stairs and round the corner into the Hearing Aid Centre.

After a short wait I was ushered into a little booth by a charming man called Adnan – not his real name (actually it is) – and given a pair of headphones and a little buzzer thing to hold. They test one ear at a time playing different sounds at odd intervals, pitching high or low, and you have to press the buzzer every time you hear a sound. The sounds are audible at first but as they get fainter you're not sure whether you've heard them or not so you just keep pressing the buzzer in case – what the heck?

However, they are used to idiots like me and can gauge a pretty accurate idea of any degree of hearing loss. Emerging from the booth I was shown a graph with bands across it indicating either stone deaf, chronic hearing loss, moderate, mild, right down to why-are-you-wasting-our-time. The little crosses on the graph indicated I had moderate to mild hearing loss consistent with my age.

Adnan explained that hearing aids would benefit me in certain situations like a noisy restaurant, but there was no immediate hurry. He said, 'I'll show you,' and fiddled about with a pair and placed them gently in my ears. Then he led me down the stairs to the main shopping floor where, thankfully, my captive audience had now dispersed. The sound just hit me like a wave.

'Is it always as noisy as this?' I asked him. 'Is it more crowded in here than usual?

'No', he replied, 'you are now hearing what I'm hearing.' Really? We were standing near a makeup counter where two girls were examining lipsticks and I couldn't believe that taking off the lid of a lipstick and putting it back again could make such a noise. Adnan reached towards me and removed the hearing aids and suddenly the room went quiet with a muted background hum rather than a cacophony of sound. Oh my goodness! I am deaf as a post! We went back upstairs and he explained about further fittings and follow up appointments and the payment structure, and the whole thing would come to around £4,000 – (What!?) – with monthly payments in interest-free instalments for the next thirty years or so as an option.

I said I'd think about it and went home. I did think about it, for at least ten seconds, and came to the conclusion that at my age, I surely qualify to take advantage of our excellent National Health Service to provide the necessary hearing aids for me. However, this can only be initiated by making an appointment with my doctor. I don't know about your particular set-up but by all accounts this is easier said than done.

You can phone in the morning on the dot of 8.30 a.m. to be told you are number twenty-three in the queue and invited to listen to the collected works of Brahms and Wagner, interrupted every ten seconds by a recorded voice telling you how important your call is which would be answered shortly. Meantime you are number sixteen in the queue. After fifty minutes you get to be number one and think 'Aha we are getting somewhere.' Wrong. You can stay at number one for a further ten to twelve minutes before a human voice – hurray – informs you that there are no appointments available for the next two months and you should call back to repeat the whole rigmarole at 2.00 p.m. How come there will miraculously be appointments at 2.00 p.m. you ask? Apparently, they release a few emergency appointments then.

I couldn't face spending the next few days on the phone so I wrote a letter to the doctor explaining the result of the hearing test and requesting some hearing aids. I handed it in to the receptionist at the surgery at the beginning of August 2016. She told me she would give it to the doctor and I should be contacted by the hospital for an appointment shortly. I guess there are many interpretations of the word 'shortly' – as in, 'your call will be answered ...' and, 'the hospital will contact you ...' By the middle of October, I still hadn't heard from any hospital, so I dropped another note in to the surgery asking politely if the doctor would follow this up.

Eventually I got a call from my local hospital arranging for me to see an audiologist on 10 November, a mere three months after my initial request. A letter followed confirming the appointment for 10 November. The following day another letter arrived from the hospital asking me to please call them to make an appointment to see an audiologist.

I phoned and spoke to a nice lady telling her I already had an appointment for 10 November. She checked and confirmed that I did indeed have an appointment for 10 November.

Roll on 10 November, I'm going to get my hearing aids.

3rd November, a letter from the hospital, 'Unfortunately we have to *cancel* your appointment for 10 November due to 'staff shortages,' (euphemism for 'wicked Tory cuts') and another appointment made for 21 November. Getting deafer, guys!

19 November, a letter from the hospital informing me that I had *missed* an appointment made for me on 14 November at 10.30 a.m. 'despite being consulted on the arrangement.' What? When? First I've heard of it. You read in newspapers about the thousands of missed doctor's appointments that happen each year – well, this is prob- ably why: because the patient didn't know they had an

appointment to begin with! Roll on 21 November, I'm going to get my hearing aids.

21 November, text message from the hospital, *cancelling* my appointment for today. No reason given. They will contact me to make a new appointment.

I'm beginning to lose the will to hear. New appointment made for 29 November at 4.30 p.m. Letter confirming this. I made sure it was still the same year and put it in the diary.

Roll on 29 November, I'm going to get my hearing aids.

I turned up exactly at 4.30 p.m. and found the audiology department. There seemed to be no one around. I eventually found a medical-looking person and explained I'd come for my appointment. She said the consultant had gone home. Fine! I triumphantly produced my letter and showed her, date: 29 November, time: 4.30 p.m. She said, 'No, this says *14.30* – half-past two, not four-thirty.' Noooo! I hadn't noticed the 1 before the 4. Oh, for goodness sake, why can't they write in English? She said, 'I thought we had a no-show earlier.' Yes, that was me. I sent an apologetic email the next day.

I won't bore you further with this saga, just to say it continued in similar vein until May the following year – nine months since my initial application – when I finally got some hearing aids. But you know what, they are fiddly, and it took me quite a bit of practise to get them into my ears. They are not the slightest bit helpful in a crowded, noisy restaurant or party as they only *accentuate* background noise, so you still can't hear what the person next to you is saying. I wore them at a meeting with about thirty people in the room, and although the speaker's voice was amplified, it had an echoing quality which was irritating so I had to remove them. The tiny batteries only seem to last for a couple of days, indicating they need changing by playing a little tune in your ear at the most inappropriate times.

It is possible to do away with the fiddly little batteries by getting your hearing aids from a private source as you just pop them into a special little gadget that charges them overnight like a mobile phone. There are also more sophisticated hearing aids that you can regulate to say, turn down background noise and increase dialogue, but this would mean going the £4,000 route. I'm saving up.

In the meantime, I have got into the habit of automatically turning on the subtitles for every programme even when they don't feature too-fast-talking American actors, mumbling British actors who think this gives their performance more authenticity, and indecipherable Scottish actors who all sound like bagpipes to me!

4

YOU *CAN* GO OUT LOOKING LIKE THAT

... as long as you don't mind overhearing remarks like:

'Did she get dressed in the dark?'
'She obviously didn't look in the mirror before she left
   the house.'
'She must have thought it was a fancy-dress party?!'
Daughter (mine) to friend catching sight of mother in
   the street: 'Oh there's my ... no it isn't.'

WHAT *ARE* YOU WEARING?

I confess I know absolutely nothing about fashion. I do not follow trends, I hate shopping for clothes and spend my life either in workout gear for my job as a fitness instructor, or trackie bottoms and a T-shirt or sweater according to the weather. Having to 'dress up' meaning a dress or skirt, which in turn means tights and 'proper' shoes as opposed to trainers, fills me with horror.

I am considered weird by my family and friends, most of whom pore over the latest fashions and seasonal must-haves in magazines, and love browsing in clothes shops or buying online. My lovely younger (both true) sister is one of them and Monday is her clothes-buying day – only to return most of them the following day – thereby designating this day as 'Take-back Tuesday.'

You would never think we were sisters as she is the polar opposite of me, being extremely smart and beautifully dressed – in the clothes she has decided to keep! She never leaves home without makeup, tasteful jewellery and immaculate hair. She inherited this sense of style from our mother who worked in the fashion department at Fortnum & Mason in London's Piccadilly until she was 83, dressing titled ladies for Ascot and visits to royalty.

FASHION ADVICE

Having confessed to my ignorance on the subject of clothes I felt I needed some advice on how to dress for my advanced age. I thought you might benefit from this as well so I consulted a fashion expert who has advised many important people over the years, published a book about how to dress well, and has many famous actress clients who rely on her to make them look good on the red carpet. We'll call her Sarah. Not her real name. She didn't want me to use her real name because, as she so sweetly put it, 'in case the rest of the book is rubbish.' I asked her to be brutally honest about some of the mistakes older people make as well as to offer some helpful suggestions about how to get it right. Her first piece of advice is to try and get the balance right: you don't want to look too old or too young. Your body changes so your clothes have to adapt as well, which means learning how to flatter your body shape without doing a complete overhaul of your wardrobe. You don't have to be trendy.

I asked Sarah to list some 'dos' and 'don'ts' as a rough guide to looking good after the last flush of menopause. Starting from underneath, Sarah stresses the importance of a good, well-fitting bra. This is essential, which means going to a specialist shop or department where a trained assistant can help you choose the correct size, both the bit that goes around you as well as the cup size. Advice from Sarah: after you fasten it at the back, lean forward so your breasts 'fall into' the cups, then when you straighten up, your bust will be in the right place. (My friend Ginny said if she did that, she would trip over them.)

Don't wear leggings. Sarah admitted her main bugbear is seeing older women wearing leggings, especially patterned ones. She begs you *not* to wear leggings with just a T-shirt or hooded top unless you are on your way to the gym or are toned and fit. Why? Mainly because with age, your legs change shape: your calves get narrower as your muscles shrink, and your knees get wider. This means that many – no, most – older women, even slim ones, develop fat knee syndrome (FKS). Look down, girl! I'm sure you had great legs when you were younger, but as with the rest of your body, things drop and droop including the flesh on your legs. A good way to discover whether you have FKS is if the bulge on your inner knee is wider than your calf; if so, you have fat knees and leggings don't look good. Even young girls have FKS when they're overweight.

I'm old enough to remember a famous British couturier called Hardy Amies who sniffily declared that a woman's knees were the ugliest part of her body and should be covered at all times. So that's why the Queen never wears miniskirts – I always wondered.

The other reason not to wear leggings is if your bottom is travelling south for the winter. In other words, it is a bit flat and droopy. Unless you do hundreds of squats every week to tone and lift your glutes – the large muscles you sit on – avoid leggings unless covered by a long top.

This doesn't mean you can't wear trousers or jeans provided they are well cut and fit nicely round your hips and bum. Don't wear the so-called 'boyfriend' jeans which are loose and baggy. Dark coloured jeans, straight leg or boot leg suit most shapes, obviously avoiding anything ripped, torn or 'distressed.' Wear them with boots or flats, not stilettos, which, in Sarah's opinion, look silly with jeans.

Do go for well-cut trouser suits from a reputable store; straight leg trousers are always safe with a blazer style jacket which always look smart especially with a silky blouse or white T-shirt. Block colours are best: black, grey, red or khaki and these will stand the test of time. You will always have something smart to pop on for an occasion or meeting.

If you're old – and how old is up to you – don't wear a miniskirt however good your legs still are. (See fat knees above.) Sarah cites, as an example, the wife of the French president, Mme Brigitte Macron, who is in her 60s and actually *hasn't* got FKS, in fact her legs are a great shape, but she does look a bit, well, awkward in those miniskirts next to the smartly dressed wives of visiting presidents like former model, Mrs Trump. Much better would be a straight skirt skimming just below the kneecap which is a flattering length for anyone whatever shaped legs you have, but make sure it's not too tight or restrictive. Uneven hems or 'handkerchief' skirt lengths look fine on young tall people, but this style on older, shorter people just looks like carelessness.

Sticking with legs, to disguise thick ankles, the dreaded 'cankles', take a tip from Cheryl Whatever-her-current-name-is and wear shoes with an ankle strap. Perversely, this does not draw attention to this area, but gives the illusion of shape. Other than that, wear trousers and blame your mother.

Do wear pretty dresses, preferably wraps or shifts. These create an illusion of a flat tummy. A printed wrap dress is especially flattering, tied at the side or back, not at the front; or choose a shift dress to hang in a straight line. Sarah advises against huge swirly patterns though, as you'll look swamped and as if the dress is wearing *you*, rather than the other way around. If something doesn't fit properly, take it to be altered, rather than hitching and pulling all evening.

A turtleneck will disguise a turtle neck, (this is like a polo neck sweater but without the rolled down bit) or a turned-up shirt collar with a little necklace nestling in the hollow of your throat diverts attention from a scraggy neck. Some women use lots of floaty scarves for this purpose. Strangely, those heavy choker necklaces seem to draw the eye to the very area you are trying to hide.

Tops with a boatneck shape at the front are flattering under a well-cut jacket. However, if you are broad shouldered and your back is a bit rounded, then avoid tops which have a low boatneck style at the *back* exposing the top of your spine where it meets the back of your neck. Unless you have the perfect posture of a dancer, it is much better to make sure the back of your top covers the top of your back – if that makes sense!

What looks dreadful, in Sarah's opinion, are those large women with massive beefy arms and shoulders who wear strappy tops in the summer baring acres of sunburnt skin – usually with baggy shorts.

And please don't dress to look sexy, begs Sarah. As if! No, she argues, she has had to advise many former models and screen stars who were used to sashaying along a cat-walk or red carpet in dresses slashed to the navel, but who have now reached the age when a similar outfit revealing acres of, even slightly, wrinkled skin above drooping boobs is, well, not a good look. This advice was reinforced by the former editor of Vogue, Alexandra Shulman, who wrote in the *Mail on Sunday*, 'No matter how pert your breasts, how great your legs, our clothes simply don't look the same as we age because they are about the person wearing them, not the items themselves. Something you wore at 30 will never look the same on you twenty years later. Clothes don't lie. There's nothing wrong with being desirable – it's just not best achieved wearing a black lace corset in public.' Ah, I must remember not to do that then!

As for colour, according to Sarah, yellow is a tricky colour to wear and looks better on dark or suntanned skin. I know that if I wear yellow people stop me in the street and offer me antibiotics! However, pale colours next to your face, something white, or soft colours like pale pink, beige or cornflower blue brings light to your face.

The ubiquitous little black dress is always a winner unless you go somewhere and everyone else is wearing one too, then it looks like a wake.

As you get older it's better to go for one classic, designer piece rather than lots of cheap, throwaway clothes, but not with some designer's name or slogan plastered across your chest – or on your belt or handbag. I promise you no one's impressed.

No halter necks (think 'arms').
No leather skirts or trousers, even black.
No bomber jackets – you're not 15.

FASHION ADVICE FOR LARGER LADIES

Following requests from some of my friends, I asked Sarah for advice on disguising the dreaded muffin top – that roll of fat that squishes over the top of your waistband – plus the notorious back fat. Yes, we've all got it.

There are various theories about what causes this: some say it's from wearing too tight trousers. This is not so. It is actually caused by your spine shrinking slightly as you get older. As you approached your 60s, 70s or 80s, you will have shrunk in height by one or two inches and the flesh which stretched nicely over your taller frame now has to go somewhere, so it settles round your middle. This doesn't necessarily mean that you are too fat. However slim you are, and I would describe myself as fairly slim, I have wodges of fat at the back of my waist that I can grab with both hands.

I asked Sarah if she would recommend 'shapewear', those elasticated garments worn under a slim-fitting dress designed to smooth out any lumps and bumps and make you look slimmer. The most well-known brand is Spanx, founded in 2000 by an American company in Atlanta, Georgia and made from nylon and spandex fabric for women and yes, since 2010, for men as well! Since then there have been many imitations and similar garments can be found in most stores.

Sarah made a face and advised avoiding these if possible because however 'light' the garment professes to be, it is still tight and restrictive and you would get increasingly hot and uncomfortable as the evening wore on, especially if you wanted to eat and drink. The only time she advises her clients to wear these is when sashaying along a red carpet in front of a phalanx of photographers snapping them from every angle. For a normal person it would be better to opt for style and comfort rather than suffer for the sake of fashion.

If only this advice had been available at the time for Cressida, 55, a friend of my daughter. Cressie couldn't resist buying a gorgeous, slim-fitting dress for the very grand society wedding of a close friend which was being held in one of those huge country mansions set in acres of nowhere.

When the hoped-for loss of ten pounds of post-menopausal weight failed to materialise, she bought an all-in-one elasticated under-garment designed to streamline her thighs, tummy and waist. All was well at first until she needed to go to the loo. A search revealed a secluded bathroom on an upper floor and she commenced the almighty struggle to pull down her tights, the elasticated horror that clung stubbornly to her torso and finally her flimsy pants. She sank down on the loo seat with a sigh of relief and a heap of clothes round her ankles when the door opened and a waiter from the catering company came in. He took one look at the aberration in front of him and hurriedly backed out again with a muttered apology, leaving Cressie mortified in mid-wee and cursing the unreliable locks on old houses. I don't know who was more embarrassed half an hour later when she came face to face with the same waiter as he proffered a tray of drinks.

I discovered for myself that wearing tights is a no-no. The waistband cuts into the flab round my middle and make the bulges even worse. Sarah advised me to try hold-ups from M&S, (but I'm sure you can get them anywhere) which are basically stockings with a lacy top lined with some sort of light rubber stuff which makes them stay up on your thigh without constricting it. I was concerned that I would be at a wedding and suddenly find them gathered round my ankles, but they are brilliant and haven't let me down once. This makes fitted dresses look much smoother.

The same advice goes for not wearing tightly fitted tops. However pretty the material, rolls of fat are not attractive (you don't say, Sarah!). If you must wear a fitted top, her advice is to pop a camisole underneath to smooth it out.

Layers look better if you're a bit plump. A tailored jacket or twinset doubles the layers and takes the eye away from the bulges. Also wearing darker colours on top like black, navy or chocolate help make the top half look smaller.

If you're wearing a belt, take it a bit lower, loose on your hips or with a blousy top. The blousiness of the top disguises the muffin area and the lower-slung belt draws the eye away from any problem bulges.

Your choice of shoes is up to you. Sarah says don't wear very high heels to compensate for the fact that you have shrunk a bit in height. These can cause your body to slump so your boobs look saggy. A slightly lower heel is better.

Another 'don't' is wearing ankle boots with skirts or dresses – they look fine on teenagers but daft on older women. Obviously, they're fine with jeans or trousers.

All fashion editors advise not being too matchy-matchy with everything the same colour or pattern. Shoes and bags don't have to match. If you have bunions, which I inherited from my mother, I can recommend a wonderful company called Sole Bliss who make lovely, fashionable shoes especially for people with bunions. Check them out if you have been suffering up to now. It's the first time I have bought shoes online and they fitted perfectly.

How do you feel about status symbol handbags? As I have already confessed my ignorance, I have to state I cannot understand why anyone would want to put their name on a waiting list for a new designer handbag costing in the region of £3,000 which won't even be available until next Spring! What's that about?! No, don't try and explain, I just don't get it. I only want to say that I have never seen a man gazing at a woman in admiration and uttering the words, 'Wow, you look amazing carrying that handbag!' Still, what do I know?

WHAT'S WITH THE HAIR?!

There are many theories about hair as you get older:

'You shouldn't have long hair over 30.' Why not? Long hair is perfectly acceptable on an older person as long as it's in a well-cut style and not looking as though accessorised by a pointy hat and broomstick!

'Grey hair looks fine when you have a young face.' But you won't always have a young face, sweetie!'

'What about a nice perm.' Noooo!

'Just to add a bit of body.' Noooo!

'A jaw-length bob suits everyone.' No. It doesn't.

'You need to trim your fringe.' No. You don't.

A lot of older people opt for a sort of hair 'hat' – channelling their inner Princess Anne – a style so rigid it doesn't move even in a gale force wind. As they used to say about Margaret Thatcher: if she fell over, she'd break her hair.

And what about hair colour? I know a lot of women 'can't be bothered with the faff' of dying their hair and just let it go grey and I can understand that. It all depends on what action you take when the first grey strands appear. Once you start tinting you usually keep going. Sometimes, having grey hair can work in your favour. A cousin of mine, Karen, worked in a huge financial corporation in the City of London. She rose through the ranks to become the first female CEO of the company at age 62. At that point she decided to stop tinting her hair dark brown and allowed the natural colour to come through. It turned out to be 'iron grey' with a touch of white at the temples and she was delighted with the look, saying it gave her a sense of empowerment and left her totally free to inhabit her new leadership role. Good for her.

For most people though, grey hair is associated with advanced age and I do feel that when you look in the mirror and see an old person looking back at you, you *become* that old person and this will be reflected in your personality and demeanour and the way you expect people to behave towards you. Sorry to be so blunt. I have my grey roots 'touched up' every five weeks and some subtle lights put through the front twice a year to give a more natural look. Thinking about it, the only time I feel 'old' is when I'm at the hairdresser, having returned to my seat after being shampooed with a towel wrapped round my head. The harsh overhead lights of the salon show up every line, crease, bag and wrinkle in the face looking back at me in the mirror. Yet once I return home with newly styled hair, I think I look younger. Deluded more like! I blame my hairdresser, James: I told him I didn't look as old and my hair wasn't nearly as grey when I first started going to him ten years ago, so it's his fault!

The following tips are vital, grey or no grey. Invest in a good cut. Find a hairdresser who has been trained in the modern way of cutting, preferably with a top London salon before decamping to become a stylist at your local 'Hair Today Shorn Tomorrow' or whatever ghastly pun some hairdressers think is trendy. There are many local salons run by older men who were at their cutting edge (ha ha) in the 1960s and are still inflicting that geometric cut on women popularised by Vidal Sassoon in his heyday. Or worse, a 'mullet' cut which is short on top and long at the sides, making you look like you have been attacked by someone on day release from a mental health institution. Hairdressing has evolved incrementally over the past twenty years and any stylist who hasn't kept up with the modern way of cutting will stay stuck in the past to the detriment of his or her clients.

Do not dye your own hair at home, especially if you are older and a bit cack-handed. You will end up with a 'block' colour and resemble Cruella de Vil. You need a professional colourist to add soft lights to break up the colour and lift your complexion. Be careful of having too many different coloured highlights though. This becomes increasingly difficult when the grey hair starts to show. Do you just have the grey roots touched up or do you have to have the whole head done every five weeks? Time-consuming and expensive.

Be aware of bed hair. I have walked behind lots of women who have 'forgotten' to style their hair in the mornings, just tidying the top bit that they can see in the mirror and leaving a flat patch at the back where they've slept.

Invest in a good pair of straightening irons. How did we survive without them for so many years?

MAKEUP

Less is more, ladies! We've all seen older women who have been heavy-handed with the makeup and look like they've been embalmed! Thick black eyeliner, sparkly eyeshadow and four coats of mascara make you look like Cleopatra-at-the-disco!

My mother, who was born in 1912, had a beautiful complexion right up to her death aged 91, probably due to her nightly liberal application of Pond's Cold Cream. By day she used a compressed foundation and powder combo called 'pancake' which she smoothed on her face with a damp puffy thing. After that went the obligatory blue eye shadow which all women used in those days regardless of their eye colour, and something called 'rouge' on her cheeks. She then took a small solid block of mascara which she used to spit on (!) to moisten before applying it to her lashes with a tiny, single bristle brush. Does that bring back memories for anyone? My mother's favourite perfume was called 'Youth Dew' by Estée Lauder. So even in the late 1920s and 30s the hidden message was, 'wear this perfume to feel youthful (and dewy?).'

I watched admiringly as a skilled makeup artist tended to a mature lady in Selfridges who applied just enough to enhance her features. When she had finished I asked her for some tips on makeup for older people. She was happy for me to use her real name for this book, but I've forgotten what it was!

She said ditch the powder. Face powder is meant to coat and make the face look matt. This is fine on young oily skin, but looks dry and dusty on older skin, which is much drier. However, she does use loose powder on eyelashes before applying mascara to make them look thicker. She used a clean mascara wand to do this, followed by two coats of mascara paying special attention to the outer lashes top and bottom.

Other advice was to be careful of sparkly eye shadow which just goes into the creases, preferably sticking with a muted beige or light grey colour. No, blue eye shadow does not bring out the colour of your eyes, it just looks dated. And don't be heavy-handed with the eyebrows – a hard pencil line makes you look permanently surprised. We all have a relative whose pencilled-on eyebrows are always asymmetrical.

Your eyebrows do get more sparse with age and, if they become practically non-existent, it is worth considering having them tattooed with semi-permanent dye. As with a hair stylist, you need to find a highly trained beautician to do this. She will use little feathery strokes of colour with a fine microblade into the upper layer of the skin which looks quite natural. This is rather expensive, but it does cut out a lot of faff and will last for at least two years.

There is not a lot you can do to disguise the bags under your eyes except to use one of those light-deflecting products which will blot out the dark circles, but make sure it is blended in properly before you add your foundation. Don't bother having plastic surgery to try and get rid of the undereye bags. It's invasive, expensive and not always successful. Three months and two sleepless nights later, they are back!

A lip pencil is essential to draw in the outline of your lips to stop the colour 'bleeding' into the little lines round your mouth. These will be more pronounced if you were a smoker in your youth. Our expert advised always using a lip brush to apply lipstick to get the best result. As for colour, rose pink is the most flattering depending on your skin tone. A dark red can look a bit hard, especially when it escapes your natural lip line and migrates on to your teeth making you look like Mrs Dracula at a hen night.

I hope this chapter has been helpful. It's getting harder and harder to maintain the status quo but dying your hair or having fillers put in your laugh-lines doesn't have anything to do with trying to look younger. It's about looking as good as you can for the age you are, which surely is the goal for us all. What it comes down to is putting on a nice outfit, looking in the mirror and saying to yourself, 'You know what, you look really good.' That's all you need. Do not add 'for your age'!

A little cautionary tale to end this section: my friend Linda took an armful of clothes into the changing room of a well-known store. She bumped into an old school friend she hadn't seen for years in an adjoining cubicle and after an initial brief catch-up chat, they started light-heartedly appraising each other's chosen outfits, being quite honest about what they thought, admiring some and giving a grimace of disapproval of others. Eventually, the school friend emerged wearing an outfit that caused Linda to shriek with horror: 'You can't wear that! It's awful; the colour is wrong, the style doesn't suit you – take it off immediately!' which elicited the frosty response, 'This is what I was wearing when I came in.'

Ooops!

5

LET'S HAVE A CHAT

When I get together with my friends we chat about various things, as I'm sure you do. The talk often turns to how the world has evolved during our lifetimes, occasionally leaving us senior citizens striving to keep up with changing attitudes and innovations and wondering whether these have improved the lives of those coming after us or not.

When my father-in-law escaped from Russia and arrived in this country in the late 1920s, the first English words he learned were 'cup of tea' which he thought was one word: 'cuppotee', always preceded by the word 'nice.' So please join me and my friends for a nice cuppotee and a chat.

CHILDREN GROW UP, IN SPITE OF THEIR PARENTS!

Have you got children? If so, they must be grown up by now like mine. I last gave birth to someone – I forget who – over fifty years ago. In fact, starting in 1959, I had five children in seven years. I didn't intend to have so many children so quickly, I just didn't realise what was causing it. (Ba-boom!)

I don't know if you remember but unlike today, when you were pregnant back then you were encouraged to eat for two. I ate for six. I must be the only person to put on weight during labour. I assumed the extra pounds would miraculously disappear straight after the birth, blindly oblivious of the fact that newborn babies do not emerge from the womb weighing four stone.

No elective caesareans or epidurals for us – in the 60s the buzz word was 'natural childbirth' and you attended classes where you were taught that breathing/panting in a specific way during contractions would ensure a speedy and pain-free delivery while you remained fully in control, sipping Champagne and having your nails manicured.

Not so. After three contractions I was demanding full anaesthesia and only to be woken when the kid started school. Breast feeding was encouraged but in my case that lasted about ten minutes before dispatching my husband to the nearest chemist to stock up on Cow & Gate powdered milk and Milton sterilising equipment.

Although we were not pampered with disposable Pampers, on the food front I do think that children born in the 60s ate more healthily than the present generation, mainly because chickens laid eggs rather than nuggets and fish had fillets rather than fingers. Even so, my children would only eat a breakfast cereal if they had seen some cartoon animal sing and dance about it in a TV commercial – or anything left under a car seat for three weeks. I predict future generations will probably be born with a mobile phone already embedded in their palm and the only way to communicate with your child will be by text: 'Dinner's ready', 'What do you want for your birthday?', 'We've moved.'

I believe children are conceived with passion, carried with indigestion and raised with love. I'm sure, like me, you gazed at your innocent little sleeping son and wondered what occupation he would go for as an adult. A doctor? No, he'd have to wash his hands. A High Court judge? No, he'd have to wear a silly wig. A Rabbi? Nah, he'd have to work on Saturdays – besides, it would help to be Jewish.

We were told never to make a child feel guilty. Why not? What's wrong with a bit of 'Never mind, I'll do it myself' or 'After all I've done for you, that's the thanks I get.' It never did us any harm – did it?

You go through all the various phases of childhood and somehow survive the turbulent teenage years during which my husband and I realised we could never get divorced because neither of us would want custody of the children! But then, suddenly, a miracle happens: your children grow up, they become proper adults and you have produced some bright, loving people who will be your closest friends for the rest of your life. What is that old saying: at age 18 your parents haven't a clue about anything; at age 21 it's amazing how much your parents have learned in the ensuing three years.

It's true, as parents you never stop learning and it's hard to step back and watch them making mistakes: dating people who you know are obviously not right for them, even allowing marriages which you know, instinctively, will eventually lead to divorce. Very few couples of my acquaintance have not gone through the trauma of at least one of their children's divorce with all the misery that entails. But you learn to keep your lip buttoned up and stay out of couples' complications and sibling skirmishes. You know that whatever you say in good faith will be taken the wrong way and you will end up the bad one. Remember the old adage: a mother's place is in the wrong. Whenever I say anything detrimental in front of my younger son, he rolls his eyes and declares he has booked me in to the Home for the Mentally Bewildered – maximum security wing!

So, you do not comment when your daughter or, even worse, your daughter-in-law, asks her children what they would like to eat, then proceeds to cook a different meal for each child. What's that about? Can you imagine if I had to do that with five children? I'd never get out the kitchen! Anyway, according to my friends it seems that their grand-children subsist on a diet of pasta or pizza. Luckily my lovely daughter-in-law is more knowledgeable about certain aspects of nutrition than I am which is probably why her two teenage children tower above me, so just shut up, Grandma! Your children are fine, your children-in-law are great, your children-in-law's parents are lovely (fortunately, mine are!) and each grandchild is a genius – sorted.

How times have changed: some for the better, some, in my opinion, not so good. Robots now deliver shopping to our doors (I hope they have the wonky left-hand wheel which is obligatory in all trolleys), our children freeze their eggs, have IVF babies, search for love online, get divorced, become paranoid if separated from their mobile phones for more than a minute, and are on-call 24/7 from their jobs. Then they wonder why they're stressed!

We older people may have baulked at first when presented with our first mobile phones and put up with the gritted teeth of our children as they strived to control their impa-tience at our inability to master the blasted thing. Some elderly people still refuse to own one which drives their children insane in case they need to get in touch with them urgently. Once we get the hang of it, though, how delighted we are at the freedom and advantages it bestows. Instead of playing 'telephone tag' with your friends, where you phone them and leave a message on their answering machine, and they call you back when you're out and so on, now you simply text, 'Meet you at Pret, 1.30 p.m. on Wednesday?' and you get a reply back within hours. Sorted!

I love my Whatsapp 'Kids & Mum' group on my mobile where I can get in touch with all my children with one text and relish the hysterically funny strands they produce in reply, each one feeding off the other, which makes me laugh out loud. If you haven't mastered how to use a computer or tablet yet, do persevere. There are courses you can take to teach you how and the pleasure you will get from YouTube videos and the ability to look up anything you want to know on Google is priceless. I am useless at word games but many of my friends communicate by playing online 'Words with Friends' which is basically Scrabble on a computer. I even Google for instructions on how to dismantle my vacuum cleaner when it needs cleaning, though reversing the instructions putting it together again can be a bit taxing. You will definitely need a mobile phone to keep in touch with your grandchildren. Talking of which (please don't take the following too seriously):

DON'T TALK TO ME ABOUT YOUR GRANDCHILDREN!

I absolutely love my grandchildren. They are bright, funny and I find them endlessly interesting. However, I don't love yours and I don't find them remotely interesting. Why then, do people assume I do? It was bad enough when we were all new grandparents and had to coo over endless photos of lookalike newborns, gushing 'Isn't she gorgeous!' while thinking 'Oh Lord, that poor child.'

It's even worse once the toddler and preschool period is past and the grandchildren are in their teens or twenties. This seems to add another dimension to the level of boredom someone can inflict on you. I was at a party and chatting with a lady and having quite an interesting conversation on a variety of topics – until the subject of grandchildren came up. Obviously, the conversation didn't go quite like this but was very similar:

> 'My granddaughter, Sarah-Jane-Louise-Whatever is just brilliant,' she told me. 'She's NVQ qualified, you know.'
>
> 'Oh really?'
>
> 'Yes, she's done hedge cutting, Facebook and modelling in Play-Doh. That's the equivalent of four A-stars.'
>
> 'That's wonderful.'
>
> 'Yes, and my grandson, Obadiah (don't ask!) is also brilliant. He's a barrister.'
>
> 'Really? Which firm is he with?'
>
> 'He's at Starbucks in Mill Hill.
>
> 'Oh that sort of—'
>
> 'And I must show you Sarah-Jane-Louise-Whatever on her gap year.'
>
> Must you?! Doesn't your heart sink when the mobile phone comes out? Flick, flick, flick.

'Here she is in the jungle with a monkey.' Flick, flick, flick 'and this is her friend with the monkey and—' flick, flick 'here's the two of them together (presumably taken by the monkey) and here she is—oh no, hang on, that's next door's dog who came into our garden and stole a burger off the barbecue. Isn't that hilarious?'

No.

I'm joking of course, but the conversation was not all that different I assure you.

I don't have any pictures on my phone. Does that make me a rotten grandmother? I admit I didn't have much patience when my grandchildren were little, although I do see the merits of having a toddler around the house – at least there is someone who can open those childproof medicine bottles and scan a document.

I remember when I was left in charge of three-year-old Gabriel and his little sister Milly (truly not their real names – they would kill me!). After ten minutes I would turn into a rap artist. The lyrics may change but the refrain was usually the same:

'Gabe, let Milly have a turn now/ don't take your shoes off/ you can have a drink if you sit nicely at the table/ put that down you'll break it/ there, you see/ don't cry you didn't hurt yourself/ shut the fridge/ if you want something ask me and I'll get it for you/ I said don't touch that knob, it turns on the washing machine/ I don't know why, it just does/ I told you not to keep opening the fridge/ and don't walk around with that glass of – leave it, I'll wipe it up/ yes, coca cola does leave a nice pattern on the carpet/ don't tread – now your socks are wet ...' And so on, usually ending in tears – mine – and leaving me in dire need of CRT (that's chocolate replacement therapy).

It does get easier as they get a bit older although I don't think I could sit through *The Lion King* even one more time: 'No the daddy lion is not really dead/ I can't help it if you've dropped your sweets on the floor/ I asked you if you wanted to go during the interval', and so on.

Some of my acquaintances seem to have much more patience. My sister was 'Grandma Monday' for one daughter, spending the whole day looking after her small grandchildren so her daughter could have a break. Then she was 'Grandma Wednesday' doing the same for another daughter. Some friends of mine insisted on going to visit their son and his family every Sunday to 'see the grandchildren.' I felt rather sorry for the son's wife having to make tea for her husband's family every weekend whether she wanted to or not.

I was warned that if I didn't bond with my grandchildren from the time they were born, they wouldn't bother with me when they were older. This has proved to be untrue as I get along with them so much better now that they're teenagers and older. I'm endeavouring to instil my love of the theatre in them by taking them to see a play or musical during each school holiday. Costs me a fortune but it's worth it when I see the joy this brings. Sometimes, as I look at my teenage granddaughter's lovely face, I can't help picturing her in a few years' time standing at the altar in a beautiful wedding dress gazing adoringly at her new husband (or wife) as the priest/ imam/rabbi intones: 'You may now text the bride.'

THE NEXT GENERATION

Depending on your age, you may also have very grown-up grandchildren. I'm talking about those in their late teens and early twenties who are apparently known as Generation Z. Why are we giving children labels all the time? They came after the Millennials (another label), those born in the late 80s up to the mid-90s. These are the ones who are often derided for being entitled and sensitive 'snowflakes' and who must be heartily sick of that description. I really admire these young people with their strong convictions about animal welfare and global warming (which is apparently my fault – well, that of my generation anyway) and the accusations abound in spite of their using hairdryers every day, driving everywhere and flying all over the world in search of adventure.

I think it is vitally important for those of my generation to keep abreast of what is going on in the lives of these young people and to keep our neural pathways flexible and adaptable, even if we don't fully comprehend what they are talking about half the time.

I guess every generation wants to rebel against the boring and conservative world order of the generation above theirs. My parents thought I was mad as I practised jiving to Bill Haley and the Comets using the door handle as a partner (anyone?). I also got the same 'Surely you're not going out looking like that?' treatment as I gave my children – though in my case it was probably because I had neglected to wear white gloves.

Although today's kids are dogmatic and intransient in lots of ways, some of their beliefs are for the best. They are virulently against smoking – which is a good thing – but their parents are terrified to drink alcohol in front of them or express any opinions about gender or race. It just makes me wonder what aspects of *their* behaviour will horrify *their* children, for it was ever thus.

My nephew, Peter, a father of four, joked that all the things he and his mates like are prohibited by his children. He visualised groups of parents meeting in secret in someone's garden shed and smoking cigarettes and drinking whisky and eating shortbread biscuits where the kids can't see them. Apparently, the latter are made with palm oil which is detrimental to orangutans. I had to get my young granddaughter to explain that one to me: the native rainforest's trees that provide the sustenance and shelter for the orangutans and species like them are being destroyed and replaced with palm trees to provide the cheap palm oil for the food industry that is causing the problem. Also, the felling of trees in Brazil, Indonesia and elsewhere is responsible for at least a third of the increased carbon dioxide superheating the earth. Who knew? We can learn so much from these children if we take the trouble to listen.

They are taller, healthier, certainly more opinionated and so much brighter than us in so many ways, yet so much more ignorant in others. For example, my husband was honoured with an OBE by the Queen, which was lovely for him, but I can't tell you the number of young people who assumed the letters after his name were part of his surname. I had a phone call from someone working in a *bank* who asked to speak to Mr Obe, and the number of letters he received from various PAs, obviously on work experience, that began 'Dear Mr Obe.' Scary!

What I do admire is their entrepreneurial acumen in using social media to earn money and the respect of their peers. I'm thinking of the young *Strictly Come Dancing* star Joe Sugg and his sister Zoella and their ilk, who have built up a fortune of many millions by broadcasting daily 'video blogs' to their fans. These clever clogs become 'influencers' (there's a new word we older people have to absorb) meaning someone who is paid both in money and goods to become, essentially, a freelance digital marketer. Apparently, it is now passé to advertise something like mascara or straightening irons via TV commercials. It's much more effective to commission young people to do it instead. You get a chatty girl to film herself making up her eyes and styling her hair whilst eulogising about the effectiveness of those particular brands, thus ensuring that her millions of followers are guaranteed to do the same. Job done! That is how they are sent freebies and paid huge sums of money by companies manufacturing clothes, jewellery and makeup to promote their wares. Well done kids – respect. High fives, or whatever!

I do hope that the generation gap doesn't mean we lose touch with each other as far as humour is concerned. My teenage granddaughter and her friends were getting ready for a night out and I said jokingly (or so I thought), 'Where are you guys going to stare at your phones tonight?' to be greeted by looks of blank incomprehension. At one time we all shared a notion of what was funny: Morecambe and Wise were funny. Even today, however many times you watch them with Andre Previn, Penelope Keith and Shirley Bassey (how she kept a straight face when her shoe came off as she sang and they replaced it with an old boot, I'll never know!) you have to laugh. I just know that Generation Z would be horrified at the sight of Benny Hill chasing scantily clad females round a park, but we knew it was just harmless fun and my generation would still smile hearing that distinctive music that accompanied the sequence. That great humourist, E. B. White, author of my grandchildren's favourite Stuart Little books, declared, 'Analysing humour is like dissecting a frog – few people are interested and the frog dies.' It seems, to my friends and me, that nowadays everybody is offended by everything. We were delighted when the #MeToo movement first broke and feel it has done a great deal more than liberate women from being controlled by powerful men. It has heralded a new culture in which women are being listened to and respected, which is great, but don't you increasingly feel that it has gone too far? By conflating allegations of relatively mild social transgressions – a friendly hand on an arm to emphasise a point – with those of more serious harassment or even sexual assault feels counterintuitive. Of course, this is only my opinion based on my generational experience but I just want to say, lighten up everyone, enjoy and cherish your relationships with your partners, colleagues and friends. Live, love and laugh because the years go by so quickly and suddenly, you're alone – and that ain't much fun, I can tell you!

I know from the many chats I've had with social workers and leaders of clubs run specifically for older people while researching this book, that many couples – and widows/ widowers – get stuck in the same old rut. Their friends either die or move away so their social circle gets increasingly narrower and they lose their sense of curiosity and spirit of adventure through inertia and boredom. Every day is the same old routine and often the only conversation they have is with the person at the checkout in the supermarket.

If you recognise yourself or someone you know, maybe it's time to shake it up a bit.

TRAVEL BROADENS THE BEAM (ESPECIALLY ON A CRUISE!)

My husband and I were friendly with a couple of similar age called Joan and Harvey. Joan and I met at a childbirth class while we were both pregnant, and saw each other socially for many years. The friendship petered out when they moved further away and also because my husband and I couldn't bear Harvey! He was one of those cold, controlling men and the marriage was not happy. Joan had always had a hankering to travel to other countries but Harvey wouldn't contemplate it, citing bogus financial reasons (he was successfully self-employed) or some feigned illness to stop Joan going on her own. Once the feigned illness became a reality and he died, I tried to persuade Joan to realise her dream and go travelling. She admitted that years of caring for Harvey during his long illness had left her too exhausted to even think about it and anyway, at 73, she was too nervous to go on her own. She had few friends because of her horrible husband and was not close enough to anyone she could ask to accompany her.

She knew it was no good asking me. I am well known amongst my friends to be weird enough to hate holidays and the thought of travelling anywhere makes me want to dive under the duvet and stay there! I haven't left the country for about fifteen years. I hear that when you get to an airport nowadays, you have to remove most of your clothes and shoes and submit to an intimate body search before they let you board – after confiscating your moisturising lotion. I don't see how anyone can concoct a bomb from a bottle of Boot's No.7 anti-ageing (that word again!) formula, but then I'm no chemist.

However, after much persuading, Joan booked to go on a cruise. She told me afterwards that once ensconced in her cabin, she sat there literally shaking with nerves and wondering what she was doing there and had she made a dreadful mistake. The first evening she was shown to a table and met her dining companions who turned out to be another widow, similar in age to herself, an older married couple and two gay men who had been partners for twelve years. She instantly bonded with the other single lady and when the ship docked at various ports, they went off together to explore the markets. Over the course of the week, however, it was the gay men who turned out to be a real comedy duo and their banter and cheeky comments about the other passengers reduced her to helpless laughter every evening. She had a wonderful time and kept in touch with her new friend and, as she told me excitedly, they planned to go on another cruise together in the summer. She was just rushing off to buy some new clothes. From being an old, drab, worn out housewife, Joan blossomed and looked ten years younger.

I'm sure there are many people like Joan who need that little extra push to expand their existing lives and branch out to explore new horizons. Travel agencies report that 70% of their bookings are made by pensioners with more than a fifth of those being women travelling solo, either to meet new people or with a friend but wanting their own room.

There is a huge variety of choice and cost from escorted tours on small ship cruises along the Croatian coast to spotting rare mountain gorillas in Uganda. There are 'special interest' holidays such as the Verona Opera Festival or music and jazz, and my friend Nadia, a keen amateur artist, flew to Tuscany for a four-day painting tutorial holiday, bringing back delightful pictures of idyllic scenery. I would encourage anyone to just get out there and do it.

My friend Dilly has her old age solution carefully worked out. When she gets too old and infirm to look after herself she has no intention of ending up in a care home. Instead, she is going to rent out her house and use the money to book herself on an endless back-to-back cruise liner. As she says, you have your own room and bathroom, food and nightly entertainment on tap and there is a resident doctor and nurse should you need medical attention. Best of all it works out far cheaper than the cost of being in a care home! What's not to like?!

I guess my aversion to holidays started when I had to drag five children to a sunny destination to break up the tedium of every long summer break in the school term. Whether in a hotel or self-catering, without my usual home comforts of a washing machine or the eccentricities of my own oven, these sojourns felt more like hard work than a welcome break. Once the kids were old enough to go off with friends or the inevitable backpacking around India, I decided enough was enough and I'd prefer to stay at home. Fortunately, my husband agreed.

If I could choose a short break I would go to New York. I love the theatre, especially musicals, and a few days of sightseeing and a different Broadway show every evening would be my idea of heaven. I don't like the sun so a pool-side holiday is not for me (think crepey chest). I know, I sound like a miserable old cow but what irks me are the constant references to food: 'What do you want to do about lunch?' 'Do you fancy a coffee?' 'Did you book a restaurant for tonight?' 'Shall we meet for a drink first?'

Honestly, I used to think if one more waiter puts one more menu in my hand – well – no wonder everyone comes home from holiday weighing 10lbs heavier.

I am definitely in the minority. Most people I know can't wait to pack and go at the drop of a hat. That includes my friend Josie and her husband Nick, who can't seem to stay at home for longer than it takes to have their clothes cleaned, before booking their next trip abroad. On their return I have to listen to Josie's tales of woe that seem to permeate every holiday: the hotel was bad, the food was worse, it rained every day, the airline lost their luggage, she fell over (wrist in a cast), *he* fell over (home in a wheel-chair), she got bitten, he got diarrhoea and so on.

'So why go?'

'Oh, we had a wonderful time.'

Okaaaay.

Please don't let me put you off. If you are stuck in the aforementioned rut, get on to a respected travel company who specialise in holidays for older people, like Saga, and see what's on offer. You'll be surprised at the variety of places to see and things to do. Go for it – you'll have a great time.

As for me, I am very happy in my home as I settle down with a nice 'cuppotee' – which I don't have to order from room service – a couple of fig rolls and Netflix.

6

'SOME PEOPLE SHOULDN'T WRITE DIET BOOKS!'

'Some people shouldn't be allowed to write diet books!' proclaimed my neighbour, Marcella, who had popped in to borrow a cup of money.

'Look at that!' She gestured towards the newspaper article I had been reading before she came in. 'That' was a serialisation in the *Health* section of the latest 'sensational' diet book, a genre of which Marcella was both an avid reader and a scornful critic. Marcella is of Italian extraction and tends to be voluble on certain matters.

'So that's yet another fifty pages of bollocks followed by a further fifty pages of so-called "delicious" recipes that nobody in their right mind would follow! See that...' she jabbed her finger at the section entitled, 'healthy breakfasts' and quoted: 'For a substantial and healthy breakfast, gently simmer six ounces of smoked haddock in water infused with herbs, peppercorns and a bay leaf for ten minutes and add a lightly poached egg on top.'

She gave a snort of derision. 'I'd like to say, "listen you prat, I've got three kids to get up in the morning, washed, dressed, fed and teeth cleaned, retrieve their gym gear and lost homework, before putting a load of washing in the machine, feeding the cat, getting myself looking halfway decent and taking them to school on my way to work. When, exactly, do you think I've got time to simmer some (expletive) smoked haddock, let alone sit down and eat it?!" Idiot!'

I kept very quiet. As the author of two previously published diet books, I didn't feel able to join in this discussion. Marcella was, in fact, quite slim having followed the advice in my latter book after her youngest, Alfredo, was born but still resorted to the occasional binge when under stress.

'Some of the books are OK, aren't they?' I ventured.

'Possibly,' she conceded, 'but most of them don't seem to have a clue about ordinary women's lives. It's much easier for men. When men become immersed in something, they can go the whole day without eating – no problem. But it's *women* who do most of the shopping, cooking, feeding children and generally dealing with food. In other words, we are surrounded by temptation all the time and that is very difficult when a child leaves one square of toasty cheese on a plate. I mean, try throwing that away when you're starving hungry.'

I tried again, 'Maybe you shouldn't allow yourself to get—'

'And they cheat!' she cried, now into full-scale rant mode, 'they show you a lovely colour picture of one of their healthy meals and you think, "Oh that looks nice and filling," then you see the caption above it: serves four. *Serves four*! A quarter of that wouldn't satisfy a mouse! And do they assume there are four people in every household all on the same diet? It's rubbish.'

After a few more grumbles about the diet industry in general, Marcella became bored with the subject and had forgotten what she actually came in for, so we had a cup of tea and she told me how worried she was about her Italian mama, who was 68 and so fat and unfit she needed help to get out of a chair. As a diet counsellor of nearly thirty years standing, could I help her in any way? I explained I could only help if the person actually wanted to do something about her weight, and as her mother still lived in Italy and couldn't speak English this might be a bit difficult. Marcella said she had tried and tried to give dietary advice but her mother refused to change her lifelong pasta/pastry and chocolate habit, washed down with copious amounts of wine from her uncle's vineyard. She also never did any exercise.

The problem with Marcella's mother and a lot of women – and men – is that they think getting older inevitably means gaining weight and they can do nothing about it. Statistics show that between the ages of 40 and 55, the average woman gains up to 15lbs and it continues to creep up during the ensuing years.

This is partly due to the decrease in metabolism which goes with muscle loss. Personally, I think it starts much earlier with extra weight gained during pregnancy which you never quite lose after the baby is born, and subsequent pregnancies exacerbate this so you never quite get back to your pre-preg state.

The menopause doesn't help either, as you have probably discovered. Your shape changes; as your level of oestrogen goes down, the circumference of your waist goes up. My friends and I still remember how in our 20s we wore flared skirts with different coloured elasticated belts to accentuate our very small waists. None of us seems to have a waist anymore, even the slim ones.

I must admit I am shocked when I go somewhere public like a museum or the theatre and see how many people, mainly women over 50, who are overweight bordering on obese. Surely they are asking for trouble especially in their weight-bearing joints like hips, knees and ankles, not to mention the strain on their hearts having to pump blood round an enlarged body through arteries and veins being compressed by fat. There are so many warnings in the press about the link between obesity and diabetes and cancer but sometimes this doesn't seem to register when faced with a red velvet cupcake. Don't get me wrong here, I'm not suggesting everyone should strive to be skinny-skinny: that looks just as bad in the other direction. Models are skinny – they are paid to be. You are not. Women who starve themselves into that extremely thin state where they appear to be 'hanging' in their trousers instead of wearing them look gaunt and strained with the effort and much older than they are. They are also in danger of developing osteoporosis.

My continuing belief is that women should be viewed as more than their dress size, whatever that happens to be. The important thing is for each person to be happy with how they look. There is a very wide window of looking 'normal' – it's called slim – to which I think most people strive to be. Any size between 8 and 16 can be classified as slim depending on your height and bone structure. You have flesh covering your bones and muscles and your clothes fit you nicely in spite of your changing body shape. It gets trickier as the years go by but you can only do your best.

So, let's get to the nitty gritty: do *you* need to lose weight? Maybe you are slim but still struggling to stay that way.

A lot of slim people still have that 'eating when stressed mentality' and try to rigidly control their eating by 'being careful.' Being careful is fine up to a point, but if you are so rigid that one slip, such as eating a slice of pizza left on a child's plate, sends you scurrying to the biscuit tin because you've 'done it now' and need to eat everything in sight so you can 'start again tomorrow' – isn't so good.

I know how difficult it is to lose weight. People sit in front of me and tell me they eat very little but the scales stick stubbornly at the same high number. If this is you, tell me: have you ever done the following absentmindedly?

- Pinched half a fish finger from your grandchild's plate
- Eaten the last mouthful of ice cream in the pot as it was melting
- 'Tidied up' the apple pie so it would fit on a smaller plate in the fridge
- Picked at the chips that someone else ordered in a restaurant

And you wonder why the scales won't go down?! Look, if you do need to shed a few pounds, please don't try any of the fad diets that proliferate in books, magazines, newspapers and online. Every new diet promises all the food you can eat, instant results and strangers coming up to you on the bus and asking you to dance. These faddy regimes simply focus your mind on the 'diet' with all the feeling of deprivation that entails. Statistics show that an extremist approach to diet and deprivation is the fastest route to failure. Most of these diets claim to be based on scientific fact, but generally, the author takes some vague 'fact' and embellishes it as a marketing tool to sell more books.

I assure you some writers of diet books are more motivated to making themselves rich rather than an exaggerated concern for your wellbeing. (Irony was never my strong point!)

Certain diets take credit for lowering cholesterol, curing 'fatty liver' disease, improving heart health by increasing circulation and actually reversing a serious medical condition like type 2 diabetes. This may be true, but it is the pounds lost that has caused this result, not necessarily the method used to do so. Many health professionals are concerned that rapid weight loss regimes can revert into rapid weight *gain* regimes over the course of several months when on the 'maintenance' phase. Does that mean all those health problems 'cured' will return with a vengeance?

Anyway, why would you want to be on a permanent diet? Surely it is better to find a way of eating that you can live with day by day, encompassing healthy food that you enjoy rather than focusing on some obscure regime? There must be some food that you like to eat other than Nutella, out of the jar, with a knife.

Let's face it: you are living in the real world here, where there are social occasions, family gatherings and holidays where you eat in restaurants or go around to your friends' houses. Are you forever going to be the guest from hell saying, 'I can only eat broccoli on Thursdays,' or 'this is my Fast day'?

Most diets work – while you stick to them. The problem, as you know, is keeping the weight off once you've lost it. If you're lucky you may have stumbled on a regime that works for you and you've managed to keep your lower weight stable, only resorting to your 'diet' every now and again when you've had a blip and gained a few pounds. Good for you.

Mainly though, for most people, following any prescribed diet devised by someone else doesn't work however many times they churn out the same book under different titles. It's a bit like putting yourself into a prison cell, handing the key to someone else and saying, 'Here, live my life for me because I'm too weak to decide for myself what to eat. Show me which "delicious recipes" I need to follow (which serve four!).' I realise that, at the beginning, you may be thankful to hand over your eating decisions to someone else but, like all prisoners, soon you want to break out of your diet cell and, when that happens, you go raving mad and eat everything in sight. Not good. You have to decide what you want. Do you want a quick fix, or do you want to be permanently slim for the rest of your life? If the latter, you need to decide what you are prepared to do to achieve that.

Let's say you need to lose 20lbs – just to pluck a figure out of the air, but one which seems to be an accurate assessment for most people. What difference would it make to you to lose that extra weight? Obviously, you would feel lighter and slimmer but what other benefit would that mean to you? Would it mean the pain in your hips disappearing when you first struggle out of bed, or being able to lift a grandchild and run around playing hide and seek? I don't think wearing a tightly fitted dress would figure for many at our age, but not looking a total fright in a bathing suit on your cruise might! What is it that would motivate you to actually persevere long enough to see your plans materialise? It's worth thinking about.

To get a sense of what this means, picture yourself feeling fat and lumpy in the corner of a room. This is the 'fat corner' and your expression is resigned and gloomy. Now picture yourself at the lower weight in the opposite corner of the room. You are looking slim, attractive, exuding loads of energy and smiling happily. This is the 'slim corner.'

How are you going to get from the 'fat corner' to the 'slim corner'? What usually happens is you decide to go on a very strict diet, allowing yourself only 500 calories a day. You proudly mentally tick off 'day one.' By day three, your head is thumping, you feel lightheaded and starving and snap at a loved one – then feel guilty. To compound matters, your printer has broken – again – you cut your finger on a piece of kitchen foil and someone drives into a parking space you were about to back into. You snap – and dive into the nearest newsagent to grab as much chocolate as you can and binge-eat for the rest of the day. What you have done is simply move away from the 'fat corner' without a concrete plan of sustainable action. Your fad diet has simply pulled you back into that corner. What you need is a plan that will allow you not simply to move *away* from something undesirable but to move *towards* something better. Do you get that? If you want to make your life better, then *you* have to make it better; no one is going to do it for you. Before you can go in the right direction, you have to stop going in the wrong direction. Before you do this, you have to know what the wrong direction is.

I've been a diet counsellor for many years, and I've seen all kinds of weight loss plans, strategies and 'science-based' doctrines recycled in different forms. Before you work out a plan to succeed, you need to figure out what works and what doesn't for you personally. Come with me and take a look at some of these diet plans you may have been struggling with in the past and I'll show you why they don't work. What follows is *my opinion* – you might not agree with everything I say and that's fine. You may have found one of these methods I write about disparagingly has worked for you, in which case don't let me detract you. For example, if you find keeping a daily tally of calories consumed is your chosen way of keeping slim, then please continue doing so. But if you have tried this – or whatever the current revamped version is – several times, and a year later are still struggling, you may need to think again. All I'm saying is, if something I write strikes a chord with you, it may save you money or time in the future, but please, don't substitute your own judgement for mine. Here are some things that *don't* work:

NEW YEAR'S RESOLUTIONS

The worst time to start a diet is 1 January, especially when there are still mince pies left over in the cupboard and brandy butter in the fridge. Statistics show that people stick to New Year's resolutions for eleven days. From a psychological perspective this makes sense. The human brain doesn't like change. Most people can make temporary lifestyle changes for a week or two but, after that, maintaining something so that it becomes a habit requires very deliberate and conscious effort. If you are still hungover from New Year's Eve, it ain't gonna happen!

THE NUMBERS GAME

Do not buy any diet books that have numbers in the title, such as those promising *Lose 10lbs in 10 Days* or *Thin Thighs in 30 Minutes*. Everyone loses weight at a different rate and if you rely on a book, or any diet, predicting a time limit for results, you could be setting yourself up to be disappointed.

Similarly, ignore any plan where you have to count things: calories, points, fat units, ounces, GI numbers – whatever. *Everyone* underestimates the number of calories they eat each day and the amount listed on food labels is often wrong. What happens if you run out of your set number by teatime? Do you 'borrow' a few calories from tomorrow's allowance or just give up counting for that day?

Dieting by numbers may work in the short term but can be confusing. Food is food. If you eat too much of whatever it is you'll get fat. Watermelon scores 98 on the Glycaemic Index, which is very high and would make it a no-no for that set of diet rules, but it has only three calories per ounce, making it one of the least fattening foods you could eat. Plus, it's helped many of my clients who fancy a sweet treat stay away from the biscuit tin. So, work that one out!

FOOD FETISHES

Some regimes advocate eating certain foods at certain times. There used to be some crackpot theory that dictated you should only eat fruit first thing in the morning because the enzyme that digests fruits apparently goes on strike around 10.00 a.m. and after that the fruit will rot in your stomach. This is obviously nonsense, as is the advice not to eat starchy carbohydrate foods after 5.00 p.m. I don't know where that came from, but I've heard several people mention this as though it's fact. According to this doctrine any bread, biscuits or potatoes eaten after the magic hour of 5.00 p.m. will go straight to your thighs. This is not based on any scientific nutritional information, but we all know that sitting with a large bowl of crisps in your lap munching your way through it while engrossed in *Game of*

Thrones will certainly not help you lose weight. That said, the best time to eat *healthy* starchy carbohydrate food, such as wholemeal bread or cereal, is for breakfast to provide fuel for your body and brain and give you the instant energy you need to function during the morning.

Similarly, food combining: there is no medical reason for not mixing protein and carbohydrates in the same meal. Your digestive system is designed to process any combination of food you put into it, in any order, and the old traditional food combos like fish and chips, chicken and roast potatoes, spag bol, eggy sarnies etc. are welded into the psyche. This is a bogus medical reason for encouraging you to eat less food.

THE ALKALINE DIET

According to its proponents, eating an alkaline diet is easier for the body because our blood pH is naturally alkaline and the typical western diet of meat, bread, dairy, sugar, coffee and alcohol allegedly leads to internal stress on the digestive and nervous systems. That may well be the case but cutting out swathes of food and living a Spartan life of vegetables, beans, nuts and cucumber will certainly make you slim (and miserable) but will have little effect on your body's blood pH.

DETOXING

You do not need to detox. Your body already has a perfectly adequate system for getting rid of any undesirable substances you care to put into it. You do not have to help it along. Medically, there is no such thing as 'getting rid of toxins.' This is a fabrication of the diet industry to persuade us that our fat reserves are full of poison and if you could just eliminate the toxins, the fat would miraculously melt away as well. Dream on! If you suffered the build-up of that amount of poison in your body, you would probably be dead.

When I was studying nutrition, I was fortunate enough to make the acquaintance of Professor John Yudkin, Emeritus Professor of Nutrition and Dietetics at University of London at the time, whose book, *Pure, White and Deadly* about refined sugar greatly influenced my thinking about my own diet and subsequent publications. He once said to me, 'If anyone mentions the word 'toxins' in relation to weight loss, you can safely disregard anything further they have to say on the subject.'

PRESCRIPTIVE MENUS

You won't follow any diet that tells you precisely what to eat at every meal: this for breakfast, that for lunch, whatever for dinner, with the obligatory page after page of 'delicious' (no they're not) recipes. You won't bother with these – you know you won't and you didn't last time, did you? They are often time-consuming and likely to contain ingredients that you don't like, don't have in your cupboard or have never heard of!

BOOKS THAT STATE FRENCH/ITALIAN/GREEK WOMEN NEVER GET FAT

Yes, they do. Some book titles can be very misleading by suggesting that people of certain nationalities always stay slim. Maybe some French or Italian people are slim, but many are extremely fat. The Mediterranean diet, widely advocated by diet professionals, is broadly healthy but it still depends on the personal choices of those who follow it. Oily fish, nuts, fruit and fresh vegetables are obviously good for you but staples like pizza, pasta, croissants, baklava? Not so much. Again, it all comes down to an individual approach to health and moderation.

EAT WHEN YOU'RE HUNGRY, STOP WHEN YOU'RE FULL

Does anyone do this (apart from Paul McKenna)? Are you telling me that in a restaurant, after a starter and a main course, you order dessert because you are *hungry* or because you just fancy it? If, at home, you have prepared a nice dinner for yourself and, as instructed, stop halfway through and ponder whether you are full or not, conclude that you are indeed full and throw the rest of it away? I think not. More likely you would think; I'm enjoying this and I'm going to finish it.

Oh sure, it would be great if we were all in touch with our bodies to this extent, but let's be realistic here. You have been programmed that it's bad to waste food so are unlikely to stop eating when there is still food on your plate and chuck it out.

EATING FOOD YOU DON'T LIKE

I recommend you ignore any regime that requires you to completely change the way you normally eat. You simply will not stick to it. If you like eggs on toast for breakfast and some diet expert tells you to eat spirulina, donq quai root and quinoa instead, sooner or later you will revert back to your normal fare because that is what you like. By all means find a healthier alternative to a massive fry-up, but don't struggle to adapt to food that you dislike just because some bossy diet guru tells you it's healthy. Not everyone likes cottage cheese and lettuce for lunch.

LABELLING FOOD

Food is not 'good' or 'bad' it is simply food. Obviously, some foods are healthier than others, but for you personally it is better to make the distinction between foods that are good for you and foods *you can't control*. For example, some people can eat a few nuts and then stop. Nuts can be a healthy protein food (without added salt or caramel coating) but if you can't limit your consumption and feel compelled to finish the packet before moving on to crisps then chocolate, it would be better for you to avoid nuts on a daily basis.

CLEAN EATING

Even the young, gorgeous looking, photogenic, self-styled diet gurus who initially advocated this phrase in their 'healthy-eating-definitely-not-a-diet' books have now disassociated themselves from it, claiming they never mentioned it in the first place! Right.

Maybe cutting out certain foods or adding a food supplement has cured someone of an illness but that doesn't mean it has any benefit from people not suffering the same illness. Of course, eating plain unadulterated food like fish, nuts, pulses and vegetables is better for you than prepared ready meals, but some of the 'facts', such as eating vegetables raw instead of cooked is more beneficial, are not true. Indeed, sometimes cooking certain vegetables, such as carrots, releases more of the vitamins it contains than trying to digest them raw.

HEALTH BARS

I have in front of me a 'healthy' high-fibre cereal bar. It is made by a reputable cereal manufacturer and is described as containing wheat bran, oat cereal and honey. Sound like a brilliant substitute for breakfast on the run – until you look more closely at the ingredients such as glucose syrup, sugar, invert sugar syrup, fructose, honey, dextrose and glucose-fructose syrup. That is *seven* different types of sugar, not to mention the vegetable oil flavourings, salt and emulsifiers. Need I say more?

SHAKES AND JUICES

Look, if you want to spend your time peeling, chopping, whizzing and blending to get a drink that you will swallow in ten seconds then don't let me stop you. I agree that juiced fresh fruit and vegetables might well be full of vitamins, but it's still devoid of all the fibre that makes them nutritious. Firstly, you are denying yourself the pleasure of tasting, chewing and swallowing proper food. Secondly, a drink doesn't engage the receptors in the jaw which react to the chewing motion by telling your brain that you have eaten and to switch off the hunger signals. It takes less time to down the drink than it does dismantling and washing the juicing machine.

Having said all that, I have to admit that my youngest daughter, who is a TV producer, makes a thick, green disgusting looking concoction for herself every day which she takes to work and sips throughout the morning whilst at her desk. This satisfies her until lunchtime so hey, go figure, what do I know?

DIET PILLS

Many people, including doctors, were delighted when Orlistat was passed by the Medical Council as safe to pre-scribe as a weight loss aid and they hastened to try it. As you know, this drug prevents your body from absorbing the fat in the food you eat. This would – allegedly – allow you to scoff as many chips, crisps and other high-fat foods as you like without gaining weight from the fat they con-tain. In theory, this should work. Many patients, however, just as hastily abandoned it when the embarrassing side effects became apparent. I won't go into details but just ask anyone who was wearing white trousers. Well, the undigested fat had to escape from somewhere!

Please don't buy diet pills over the internet. Some amphetamine-type pills are still available but are no longer prescribed in this country because they were found to cause medical problems; just trivial side effects like heart disease and kidney failure. Don't – it's not worth risking your long-term health.

VITAMIN TABLETS

Just as you don't need to waste your money buying diet pills, the same applies to vitamin tablets, although most people take vitamin C as a precaution as they believe it will prevent them catching a cold. It won't. Eat an orange instead. You would have to have an extremely bad diet not to get all the vitamins and minerals your body needs – unless you've jumped on the vegan band wagon in which case you will probably be deficient in vitamin B12. Most additional vitamins taken in tablet form will not be absorbed by your body and will simply be excreted. The only vitamin I would advise taking is vitamin D which is actually a hormone synthesised by the sun. As we don't get enough sunny weather in the UK, most people are deficient in vitamin D but, as with all vitamins, you only need the lowest amount daily to be sufficient for health needs. The current trendy practice of having vitamins infused directly into the bloodstream via IV drips into a vein is not something I would recommend. Although deemed to be safe as it is performed in clinics by doctors and nurses, this practice won't make you healthier and you could be risking infection.

COLONIC IRRIGATION

I believe this is a terrible abuse of your body. Certainly, don't believe all you read about the so-called benefits. Some food, like red meat, does take longer to digest than other food but the residue does not linger in the bowel and is eliminated naturally. Sorry to be so graphic, but during colonic irrigation what you are having forcibly removed from your bowel is not only faeces, but the healthy bacteria and protective mucus that line your colon and prevent toxins being absorbed into your bloodstream through the walls of the colon. If you do this on a regular basis you could become overly constipated as your body 'forgets' how to go naturally. Not a good idea and it does not aid weight loss.

SLIMMING TREATMENTS

Don't be conned into having expensive treatments which claim to 'break down fat.' You cannot break down fat from the outside. Are you getting that? I repeat, you cannot break down fat from the outside: you can pummel it, dig needles into it, encase it in tight bandages and plaster it with mud, wax or raspberry jam: it will make no difference. Electric shocks, or having your fat squeezed between two rollers, will make you bruised and sore but will not permanently reduce the dimension of your thighs.

The beauty industry considers the phrase 'getting rid of cellulite' to mean making the skin on that area of your body look temporarily smoother, not slimmer. The only proven external method of fat loss is liposuction performed by a plastic surgeon, but this is invasive surgery with all the risks that go with that and, even then, the results may not be up to your expectations.

I have not included slimming clubs in the list of 'things that don't work' because I know a lot of people who attend regularly and have managed to keep their weight off by employing one method or another. Unfortunately, we all know people who have joined their local club multiple times yet are unable to make it work. This includes most of the people who come to me as clients.

The problem with slimming clubs is that everyone starts off with such good intentions, turning up for the meetings every week, getting weighed and applauded and receiving a badge for every small success. Seeing the same people there week after week, you form a little gang all intent on the same goals, which is a good start.

The trouble begins when you have lost an initial few pounds and the 'reward' mindset kicks in. You and a few of your gang decide that after the meeting, you all go out for a meal and order something you've missed on your diet, like fish and chips or tiramisu (why is it always tiramisu?). After all there is a whole week before you have to get weighed again and if you're careful for the rest of the week.... Uh-oh! It's the beginning of the slippery slope when your focus drifts a bit, and if you've had a 'bad' week, you decide to miss the next meeting to give yourself a chance to 'get back on track' before the following one. This might happen – the first time – but gradually, life intrudes and there are a million reasons why you can't stick to your diet and eventually the meetings go by the board. You're back to square one and have regained all the weight you lost and then some.

Never mind, when you're ready you can re-join and you'll be welcomed back with open bingo wings, and the whole process will start all over again. I personally know someone who has joined Weight Watchers nine times and still has a large tummy (not mentioning any names, Dilly!).

I've been harping on a lot about what doesn't work when you're trying to lose weight, so what does work? Hang on, I'll tell you – but for starters you need to have a plan: a goal without a plan is just wishful thinking.

When a client first comes to see me, once she stops telling me about all the diets she's tried that haven't worked, I feel I should point out a few facts:

THERE AIN'T NO FAIRY GODMOTHER

No one is going to come along and wave a magic wand to make your fat disappear. *You* put it there and only *you* can make it go away, if you want to.

IT WILL TAKE TIME

Everyone who embarks on a weight loss regime wants that fat gone – like *now*. It doesn't matter how long it took to pile on the pounds, they want instant results. Why? What's the rush? Are you planning to team up with a hot young chef to present a television cookery programme? Are you auditioning to be a pole dancer in a nightclub? What?

YOU DID NOT PILE ON THE FAT OVERNIGHT

You didn't go to bed one night weighing eight stone and wake up the next morning weighing eleven. It took weeks or months to acquire that extra layer and it will take time to disperse. So? What are you doing for the rest of the year while you lose the weight? You will still be living the same life, same family, same friends, same job if you still work – only slimmer. There is no hurry.

There is another reason why it's inadvisable to lose weight too quickly. There has been much in the press about rapid weight loss, which might work for a younger person but for the over 60s this is not the right approach. Even a moderate weight loss of 20lbs will leave you with a gaunt look on your face and saggy skin on your arms, thighs and torso. Take it slowly, one day at a time to allow your skin to 'catch up' with the diminishing fat underneath it.

YOU CAN'T EAT FATTENING FOOD EVERY DAY

Every dieter tries to factor some of their favourite fattening food into their diet each day by assigning 'points', 'allowances' or a 'treat' to it. This doesn't work for most people long term. The fact is, if you eat fattening food every day you will get fat – even if each one has 'only' 150 calories. Some days you may be able to stick to your two square chocolate 'treat'; on other days when you're a bit stressed you will eat the whole bar, then think 'What shall I eat now?'

SOME PEOPLE CAN EAT ALL THEY LIKE AND NOT PUT ON WEIGHT

True. We all know people who are naturally slim and eat whatever they like, whenever they like and how much they like, with no repercussions. They just don't think about it. Sadly, that is not you – or me, for that matter. Well, ain't life a bitch! So whatcha gonna do?

YOU HAVE FREE CHOICE

Any time you find yourself eating something you hadn't intended and saying to yourself it was because 'I was so tired' or 'I needed something sweet' or 'she went to all that trouble to prepare it' you are simply making excuses. 'It is difficult at the weekend'; 'I have to have chocolate biscuits in the house for the grandchildren' – come on now!

I know it sounds a bit harsh, but you are the only one who puts food into your mouth. No one is holding you in a headlock and stuffing chocolate brownies into your mouth. You have free choice every time. The only way to be permanently slim and healthy is to change your thinking and regain your power. The phrases you use such as those above and things like 'I can't stop eating' and 'I can't resist' make you seem powerless in the face of food. Once you start thinking of yourself as a strong person, you regain your power and become in control of your eating. Then your extra weight will go and, more importantly, stay gone. I'll show you how in the next chapter.

7

You don't take orders from a biscuit

Be careful when you're eating out
Don't let it end in sorrow
For what is in your hand today
Will be on your hips tomorrow
This isn't rocket science
You don't have to belong to Mensa
Just stock your fridge with healthy food
And thank God for Marks & Spencer.

(Memo to self: don't give up the day job.)

When I started writing this book, I had no intention of turning it into another diet book. You would think by the age of 60+ most people would know what to eat to keep themselves slim and healthy. A quick walk through any town or visit to a restaurant will show this is sadly not the case.

Recently so many people have told me they are trying very hard to lose weight but it is simply not happening and complaining they just have to look at the dessert menu to put on 2lbs. So, let me take a quick chapter to set you on the right path.

In my job as a diet counsellor, I teach people the secret of how to live like a slim person. This is not a diet. It is a way of eating that you can live with for the rest of your life. There is no 'diet' phase followed by a 'maintenance' phase – which usually means going back to the way of eating that made you fat in the first place.

The way I work is by getting into people's heads and changing the way they think about food. I do not hand out diet sheets nor suggest 'healthy' meals or, God forbid, recipes! How do I know what you like to eat? Everyone is so different with different tastes and lifestyles. Awareness is the key.

This method is the equivalent of someone teaching you how to drive a car; once you have learned how to drive, you can't 'unlearn' it. You can decide *not* to drive for a while (go back to your old way of eating) but you know you can climb back into the driving seat any time you want.

So, let me introduce you to: **The 6 – 1 Diet** ... Ta Dah!!! Oh, what's that, you may ask? On this diet, do you fast for six days and eat normally on the seventh? Noooo. So, you eat normally for six days and fast on the seventh? Noooo. You don't fast at all! Yay! What is it then? You follow your normal way of eating with some healthy modifications for six days and on the seventh day you eat your trigger food. What is your trigger food? Ah – you tell me! A trigger food is the food that made you fat in the first place and is keeping you fat now. You know what that food is.

For some people it is stodge: crusty bread, rolls, bagels – anything starchy and chewy they can pile with butter and various toppings. Pizza and pastry fall into this category. For others the choice is salty 'picky' foods like crisps, salted nuts, olives, chips dipped in ketchup. Still others, it is sugar: cakes, biscuits, chocolate, creamy desserts, ice cream etc. Alcohol is also included in this category.

Which of those food groups do you identify with? (Shut up Dilly, with your 'all of the above!') If you're not sure check out the following:

- Do you sometimes crave this food even when you're not hungry?
- Once you start eating it, do you find it difficult to stop?
- Is this the food you reach for when you're stressed, bored or anxious?
- Have you ever eaten this food instead of a meal?
- Is this the food you tried to give up when you went on a diet in the past?
- Is this the food you are definitely eating when the weight goes back on?

So, you know which food is keeping you fat. I know you know.

When I first start with a client, I explain my very simple philosophy: if you want to be slim, then stop eating the sort of food that makes you fat. By cutting out one food that is keeping you fat, it leaves you free to eat all the other food that you enjoy – which is *everything else*. Makes sense to me.

When my first book, *Stop Bingeing!* was published many years ago, that was my theme: find your trigger food and cut it out of your life. However, this made some clients burst into tears and wail, 'Does this mean I can never have chocolate ever again? Waaaah!' Of course it didn't mean that. I was suggesting that they ask themselves whether they would be prepared to abstain from ingesting Cadbury's Dairy Milk (the best chocolate in the world) for that *one day*. The following day they could ask the same of themselves – and so on.

Every client agreed that was doable and we took it from there. All these years – and literally hundreds of clients later – I have softened my approach. What I am suggesting now is that you eat 'normally' – we'll discuss what that means in a minute – on six days of the week and allow yourself to have your trigger food on the seventh day. How does that sound?

Will that help you lose weight? Yes, but first you have to:

MAKE THE COMMITMENT

If you really want to become a slim person, you have to make the commitment to *be* that slim person. This has to be a serious, conscious decision – not 'it would be nice' or 'I'll try.' 'Trying' always leaves a loophole for failure; 'Well, I tried, it didn't work.' You need to say to yourself, 'This extra weight is having a detrimental impact on my health, my energy levels, and the way I see myself. I am willing to commit to a plan to change it.'

Being slim isn't free – there is always a price. You have to decide what is more important to you: either you eat the food that makes you fat every day or you cut out that food for six days and only eat it on one day a week. I know, I know, everything in moderation blah blah, and logically, you should be able to eat a couple of biscuits and then stop. But logic and reality are two different things. If you're the sort of person who uses food for comfort and biscuits are your thing, once you get the taste you will want to go on eating.

I'm not advocating cutting out huge swathes of food like wheat, dairy, gluten, meat, alcohol, tea, coffee etc. Just the one food that acts as a trigger for you to go on eating for the rest of the day. If there is a certain food you can't control, then that food is controlling you, which may seem ridiculous but it's true.

However, there is one substance that is present in so many foods that we need to break it down a bit:

LET'S TALK SUGAR

When I suggest cutting out sugar for six days I mean 'refined' sugar that is found in all the foods mentioned above. When I wrote about this for a magazine article, some woman complained to my editor that I was contradicting myself because I encouraged people to drink milk which contains lactose – a milk sugar.

So, let's clear this up. The type of sugar found in dairy, fruit, vegetables – including sweet potato, beetroot and peas – is attached to fibre and other compounds and these are fine to eat every day. The aforementioned chocolate is full of added sugar, fat, cocoa, caffeine, theobromine and phenylethylamine – all to produce that smooth, rich creamy texture that, according to psychologists, many women find deeply sensual. Really? Personally, I don't get turned on by a large Curly Wurly but other clients have concurred with the psychologist's diagnosis.

You may have read before that sugar is an addictive substance in that it stimulates the 'reward paths' in your brain the same as heroin and cocaine. This is true. (Some dietary experts have tried to dispute this fact but they haven't met my friend Dilly, or me!) If you try and control it by having a little sugary treat every day, you will be fighting hunger and cravings *all the time*. A recovering alcoholic doesn't allow themselves to have a small sherry at teatime.

Choosing *one* of your favourite sugary treats to have *once* a week should dispel that 'deprivation' mindset and be easier to stick to. I will use chocolate as an example of the main source of sugary foods that clients find so difficult to control.

TRIGGER DAY

Just for the sake of explanation, let's call Saturday your trigger day. This is usually a family oriented or social day and therefore leaves you more open to temptation. Like some of my clients, you may have several trigger foods so, on this day, you choose just one and give yourself permission to have as much as you like of that *one* food.

If your choice is chocolate, then have a bar after lunch and another bar in the evening if you like, and then stop. This doesn't mean you then raid the biscuit tin or gravitate on to crisps and pizza washed down with sugary cola. There has to be an element of control here.

The fact that you are only eating your trigger food on Saturday makes it easier to control any cravings during the week. You just tell yourself, 'wait until Saturday.' This gives you something to look forward to rather than castigating yourself for indulging in something all the time that you know is fattening and detrimental to your health.

Here are some examples from other clients. I won't name them as I occasionally have celebrity clients and they might recognise their personal triggers:

Client one: Crusty bread. Every Sunday (her trigger day) morning she buys fresh bagels from her local bakery and eats three with butter, mashed hardboiled eggs or smoked salmon. That satisfies her stodge quota. She doesn't eat bread during the week but still has cereal for breakfast.

Client two: Cheese. Unable to resist breaking off a chunk and eating it every time she opens the fridge, she limits herself to this once a week and eats as much as she likes, including pizza.

Client three: Ice cream. She will eat a whole large tub while watching her favourite TV show in the evening of her chosen day.

Client four: Creamy cakes. She will buy a whole cheesecake and eat at least half of it during the day. The other half goes in the freezer for the following week. She will only eat fat-free dairy foods for the rest of the week, skimmed milk, low-fat yoghurt and whole-fat cottage cheese (which is low in calories anyway) etc.

Client five: Crisps. I don't need to tell you what she does!

Other clients choose one of the following as their trigger treat: wine, biscuits, pasta in a creamy sauce, roast potatoes, Yorkshire pudding with gravy.

If that is your trigger day sorted, what about the rest of the week? If you want to lose weight there has to be some modification in the food you choose. The food suggestions I mention below are simply that: suggestions, not rules for you to follow. I don't know what you like to eat. For example:

CHECK YOUR STARCHY CARBS

Let's look at carbohydrate foods like bread, potatoes, rice and pasta. These foods don't contain a lot of nutrients, or as much fibre as vegetables, but react in the body the same way as refined sugar i.e. they make you hungry and encourage that 'what shall I eat now?' mindset. You do need carbs for a balanced diet and the most beneficial time to eat them is in the morning for breakfast. Wholemeal toast or an unadulterated cereal like Shredded Wheat or porridge will give you the best start to the day by providing fuel and energy to your muscles and brain. Decide to cut out potatoes, rice and pasta for two months and see how you feel.

PROTEIN AT EVERY MEAL

You know which foods contain protein: milk, yoghurt, fish, chicken, turkey, eggs, cheese, nuts etc. Protein reacts in the body to get rid of hunger and sustain the feeling of fullness for longer. It also stimulates the production of certain hormones that raise your metabolic rate so the food you eat gets burned up for energy and not stored as fat – as opposed to sugary foods which encourage your body to store fat. Therefore, try and include some sort of protein at every meal, such as milk with cereal for breakfast or eggs. Lunch could be chicken or tuna salad, and for an evening meal, choose some other kind of protein such as beef, lamb or any type of fish with unlimited vegetables.

VEGETABLES ARE YOUR FRIEND

Fill up on raw or cooked vegetables at any time. Maybe make a little afternoon snack for yourself with raw carrot sticks, cucumber and celery with a hummus dip. Have two or three different coloured veg with your evening meal: broccoli, carrots and sweet corn make a colourful rainbow on your plate. I know things like peas and sweet corn come under the label of 'starchy carbs' with some diet purists, but I want you to feel free to eat a wide variety of foods during the six days as long as they don't contain actual refined sugar. By the way, have sweet potatoes instead of the ordinary kind as they contain less starch.

FRUIT

Clients ask, 'Can I have as much fruit as I like?' Answer: not to the exclusion of everything else. By that, if you think you will lose weight by just having an apple for lunch, you will be starving later and dive into something fattening. But a planned snack of a couple of pieces of fruit such as a small banana and some strawberries with a plain yoghurt or cottage cheese at teatime is ideal. All berries are particularly good for you.

ALCOHOL

This is a personal decision only you can make. Obviously, I don't know how much alcohol you drink, but you know it contains a lot of calories and because it slips down without your noticing, you may not realise how much it's contributing to your weight. Even if this is not your trigger, most clients just limit it to when they eat out in a restaurant or just at the weekend. Up to you.

EAT REGULARLY

Do not skip breakfast. There is a reason it's called 'breakfast.' After fasting during the night, your blood sugar levels are very low. Your body and brain need glucose to function properly and if you don't eat in the morning you will be running on adrenaline, the stress hormone from the adrenal glands. In other words you are energising yourself via stress and agitation, which is exacerbated by coffee and which will eventually set up a craving for sugar. Even if you can't face food first thing in the morning and wait until 10.00 or 11.00 a.m. before eating solid food, that's OK. People who think missing breakfast is a good way to lose weight have been found to eat much more at lunchtime and for the rest of the day. Personally, I can't go for long periods without eating – or at least a hot drink – as it makes me lightheaded, shaky and irritable.

After breakfast, count forward roughly three hours and have your lunch then. Three hours after that, have an afternoon snack then a healthy protein and veg dinner later.

Choose foods that steer your meals in a sequence that fits your personal schedule. Make it a habit to eat each meal within a certain half-hour time frame, for example, lunch between 12.30 and 1.00 p.m., afternoon snack between 4.30 and 5.00 p.m. If you eat every meal at roughly the same time each day, you'll find you only get hungry at those times and will not experience any cravings in between.

I realise that people have busy lives and you can't always eat at set times but do try and organise it if you can. Your body likes regularity, which is why you sleep at night and are awake during the day. You need to feel alert, active and ready to go in the morning, composed for an afternoon of concentration and relaxed enough to wind down in the evening. My last book was called *Only Fat People Skip Breakfast*. Need I say more?

LEAVE A GAP

Try and finish your evening meal by a certain time and don't eat anything after that until the next morning, apart from any (non-sugared) drink you like. I can't pinpoint an exact time as everyone is different, but research shows that your body will perform best and be healthier when you limit the window you eat in to align with your circadian rhythm (your sleep/wake cycle). Leaving at least a twelve-hour gap overnight is a proven way to turn your body into a fat burning machine – and you'll find you sleep much better.

I've found with clients that snacking throughout the evening is the main vice preventing the scales from going down; the picking of nuts, fruit, chocolate or biscuits, either through stress or boredom. Have a substantial evening meal and then *stop*. A trick some clients use is cleaning their teeth after their evening meal which signals the end of the eating day.

PLAN AHEAD

Do take a few minutes to plan what you are going to eat the following day. Some clients find it is useful to write this down for a few days as it helps them stick to their plan. Some can't be bothered but most clients claim this is the one thing that made the difference. Jot down what you intend to have for breakfast, lunch, afternoon snack and evening meal. Be very precise and include food you enjoy. If you're planning to eat out, you know roughly what sort of restaurant you are going to, so choose the healthy option as far as possible.

HAVE THE 'RIGHT' FOOD IN THE HOUSE

To succeed in living like a slim person, you need to have a constant supply of the 'right' food in your cupboards, fridge and freezer. As well as frozen vegetables, keep portions of cooked chicken, salmon, smoked salmon in the freezer, as a standby for when you haven't got time to shop. These protein foods defrost fairly rapidly in time for a healthy lunch. Tins of tuna and chickpeas are useful to mash into a salad, as are hardboiled eggs.

Don't be afraid to use salad dressings or sauces to make food tasty even if they do contain a bit of sugar or honey. One bar of Toffee Crisp may 'start you off' but you're hardly likely to use a whole bottle of honey mustard dressing on your salad so don't be too rigid about it.

Do be open to new ideas and different foods. There is a whole world of different food out there just waiting for you to try. It's so easy to get stuck in a rut, convincing yourself 'I always need to finish a meal with something sweet.' Well, make the 'something sweet' a juicy peach rather than a creamy dessert. I will tell you a trick that those of my clients who have the same problem use: they buy those huge Medjool dates and put them in the freezer. For their end-of-meal something sweet, they slowly nibble *one* of those straight from the freezer and swear it tastes just like toffee. It does – I've tried it. You're welcome.

EAT S-L-O-W-L-Y

I know – you have so much to do and you promised to collect the grandchildren from school today and it's always rush, rush, rush. Stop and make time for your meals, even if you have to get up a bit earlier or prepare something beforehand.

As you get older, indigestion and heartburn can become a problem and everyone I know, apart from myself, is taking Omeprazole or other proton pump inhibitors to protect the stomach lining. You really do need to sit down and eat slowly, pausing for a few minutes when you've finished to allow the food to be digested. It takes 20 minutes for the brain to realise there is food in your system and to turn off the hunger signals. If you eat too fast, you will be ingesting a lot more food until this happens. I'm not suggesting you sit for that long of course but do consciously slow down and enjoy every mouthful instead of seeing how quickly you can finish and move on to the next thing.

JUST DO TODAY

You can only do one day at a time, one meal at a time. You can't 'un-eat' what you ate yesterday, and you can't eat what you're going to eat tomorrow at this moment. Plan for the day and stick with your plan.

As each day goes by, eating this way becomes a habit and your craving for your trigger food diminishes. Just knowing you can have it on your trigger day takes the urgency out of it and, surprisingly, when it comes to that day, you might not even bother eating that junk. It happens – truly! It's what you eat on a day-by-day basis that determines what you look like and as the weeks and months mount up you will find your weight going down steadily and consistently. Tell yourself 'Just do today.'

THE SCALES

Don't be ruled by the scales. You do not need to step on every day. Whatever you weigh, that's what you weigh. It's neither good nor bad, it just is. There is no point in knowing exactly to the half-pound what you weigh all the time – you do not walk round with this number tattooed on your forehead! Therefore, don't allow this mechanical object on the floor to dictate how you feel and whether you are a worthy person or not. Some days you will feel lighter, other days a bit bloaty. Just stick with it, you'll be fine.

YOU ARE FREE TO CHOOSE

People tell me that they feel compelled to eat sometimes: 'She put this huge slice of homemade cake in front of me, what was I supposed to do?' Let me ask you: suppose you were diabetic and you knew that cake would send you into a coma, would you meekly eat it? Of course not. I realise you wouldn't want to make a fuss but you can always come up with an excuse, 'I'm really full right now, I had an enormous lunch', or 'It looks delicious, I'd love to take a slice home.' Handle it.

The truth is, whatever the circumstances, *you always have a choice*. I know this is difficult to hear but once you get it – that you are free to choose what you eat, and how you behave, and that you don't have to be influenced by other people – it's like a weight has been lifted off your mind (and, eventually, your hips).

EATING IS A LEARNED RESPONSE

Get to know yourself and how you tick. Past behaviour is a reliable predictor of future behaviour. You eat the food you are used to eating at the times you are used to eating it. Check: when is your 'high risk' time of day? For most people it's teatime when they settle down with a cup of tea to watch 'The Chase' – or do you prefer 'Pointless?' If you always have a chocolate caramel wafer biscuit (made with palm oil!) at that time, your body will come to expect that and set up a craving. To change a fattening habit, you need to identify your own pattern of eating and have a plan to counteract these crave times. Save the chocolate biscuit for your trigger day and have an apple and a yoghurt on the other days. Soon you will find yourself looking forward to that. You have changed one habit for a healthier one.

LOSING WEIGHT STARTS IN YOUR MIND

It is the thoughts you put in your mind that determines what you eat, when you eat and whether you eat something fattening or not. That's what I meant when I said earlier that I work by getting into your head and changing the way you think. Control your thoughts and you control your weight. That means, you don't say to yourself 'I can't eat chocolate because I'm on a diet', you say 'I *can* eat chocolate, I can eat whatever I like but I'm *choosing* not to eat it – *today* – because I know that it screws me up.' That is free choice, not a self-imposed deprivation. Do you get the difference?

Change the way you think about food. Don't think of that creamy cheesecake as 'delicious' – tell yourself it's just a lump of fat that will go straight to your thighs. Once you think of it that way, it loses its appeal. You're not on a diet here, you're simply making healthy food choices.

DEAL WITH CRAVINGS

Let me dispel a myth here: that if you cut out your favourite daily treat – I keep referring to chocolate as my example – you will crave it and binge. Wrong. I promise you it's much easier not to have any than to try and limit it; just having a small teaspoon of chocolate mousse when you know there is a whole bowl there. That is hard. Save it for your trigger day. I'd advise not keeping your trigger food in your home but buying it on the day you plan to eat it. No, he doesn't need it either! If other members of your family object to the removal of a certain food you wish to avoid, put it in a very high cupboard so they have to climb up on a chair then up on the work surface to get it. If you keep it nearby, however motivated you are to begin with, you may give in to temptation if you're having a stressful day.

If a midweek craving does strike, practise the three second pause: Ask yourself: 'Do I really want this? If I eat it how will I feel later? Will it be worth it?' This allows you just long enough to answer 'No' to numbers one and three. Sometimes the answers to one and two may be 'Yes' and 'Sick' – but that's your problem!

It's also good to have a planned task to do when you feel a bit niggly: tidy your makeup drawer, get out the house and go for a walk, play Sudoku or do a crossword, phone a friend for a chat. My friend Adele practised the last one every day, talking to friends for hours on the phone. She is now slim – and divorced.

A craving is a feeling, it's not an order to be obeyed. It is just a moment when you decide whether you are going to eat that fattening thing or not. That split-second decision will determine what you do for the rest of the day and how you feel about yourself. It can be an 'Oh sod it!' moment or a moment where you say to yourself, 'I'm not eating that stuff today.' You don't take orders from a biscuit! Cravings last for twenty minutes then they pass, and if you don't give in, you will be so relieved later.

THINK YOURSELF SLIM

The important thing is to have a constant picture in your mind of yourself as a slim person. I know this is difficult when you look in the mirror and are confronted with rolls of fat round your middle, but everything you do is based on your perception of yourself. As with thinking of yourself as old, if you think of yourself as fat, that is how you will mentally 'see' yourself and it will be difficult for you to implement any change. If you want to be slim, you have to pretend you are slim already and behave as if this were true – in the way you hold yourself and the way you walk, with your head up and your shoulders back, and the food choices you make.

Success doesn't just happen by chance, it's a decision. This means you may have to be a bit assertive in your old age! By which I mean learning to say 'no' when people offer you food or drink that you don't want. It means knowing you have the power to live your life as you want and not what other people expect of you. Knowing that you have the strength to succeed at whatever you set out to do.

So here it is in a nutshell (sorry!) These are ten little tips that I hand out to my diet clients. If they click with you, please write them out and stick them on your fridge. I hope they will help you make the right choices to achieve the shape you want to be – because you're worth it!

1. On a day to day basis, don't eat obviously fattening food.
2. Eat regularly – watch the clock – don't let more than four hours go by without eating.
3. Plan ahead: flash through your mind where you will be and what you will eat.
4. Always have plenty of the 'right' food readily available in the house.
5. Take a snack with you if you will be away from home for several hours.
6. Don't seek out your favourite food in shops or at parties: cravings start with your eyes.
7. Have a phrase ready for when you're tempted by your trigger food, 'I am more important than food.'
8. Don't pick – *ever*. Think of your fingers as 'weapons of mass consumption.'
9. Talk to yourself in a positive way all the time, e.g. 'You handled that really well.'
10. Constantly remind yourself why you're doing this; remember how awful you felt when you were fatter, and your clothes were tight. Feeling slim, positive and liking yourself is more important than eating chocolate.

P.S. If all else fails you could always try the Tranquillizer Diet: that's where you take four Valium tablets before each meal. It doesn't make you eat less but most of it falls on the floor! That was a *joke* people! Don't do that!

P.P.S. When you get to age 90 you can eat whatever you like, whenever you like and as much of your trigger food as you like – if you can remember what it is! You're welcome xx

8

Get off your butt!

'I didn't manage to get to the gym again today', sighed my friend, Dilly, 'that makes five years in a row.'

Much as I love my friends, I find a lot of them have the same attitude as Dilly and try and come up with every excuse under the sun to avoid doing any exercise.

We've all reluctantly agreed that getting old is inevitable. While life expectancy averages 82.9 years for women and 79.2 years for men, according to Age UK many people only remain healthy up to 65. After that the risk of heart disease, dementia, stroke and cancer rises, leaving millions facing spending the last fifteen years of their lives in a state of ill health. Not good.

That is why, increasingly, scientists are focusing on 'health span': the number of years lived in good health, the idea being to find ways to extend those healthy years. The obvious goal – to me anyway – is to be as healthy and free from pain and illness for as long as possible during my latter years. I really believe in quality of life over longevity. If you feel the same way please take heed of Auntie Lee's formula: follow the diet suggestions for making healthy food choices and keep your body as fit and strong as possible with exercise to stave off pain and stiffness.

Fortunately, over the last decade there has been a marked increase in the number of people joining gyms and doing some form of exercise. For many older people, though, the word 'exercise' conjures up visions of heaving sweaty bodies, contorted limbs, inflated health club subscriptions and exorbitant osteopath bills. They probably think Abdominal Crunch is a breakfast cereal. Please don't buy into that and, just as you ignore the latest fad diets, please dismiss books and articles in magazines written by fitness gurus, who advocate extensive exercise regimes set out in a daily routine of moves for you to follow to get a body like theirs. These are written by professional trainers who do nothing else except charge their elite clients £300 an hour to run around Hyde Park and be pictured in the Daily Mail. They assume you also have nothing else to do each day but to spend at least two hours working your body. You don't have to, even for the desired 'beach body', whatever that is.

Having said that, recent research has proved that exercise, if you put your heart into it and put in the hours, may fend off many diseases that older people suffer from. According to data from 39,700 people, things like walking, swimming, lifting weights or squats are just as effective at lowering blood pressure as taking beta blockers or ACE inhibitors. Exercise also keeps you younger for longer. One way it does this is by slowing the decline of your telomeres. These are the tiny caps on the end of your DNA strands that tend to shorten and fray with age. This leaves the DNA subject to greater risk of mutation as your cells divide and replicate.

Therefore, if you want to slow down the years, please check out the local gyms or health centres in your area. There are usually council run classes in every town as well as individual classes in church halls. You should get a reduced rate because of your age, so it won't be expensive. And don't imagine you will be the oldest one there. You won't be, I assure you.

In most areas there are venues offering a particular regime, such as a Pilates studio that uses specialised equipment, or a Spinning Club using stationary bikes. I would suggest joining an organisation that has a wide variety of classes to choose from so you can try out a couple and see if anything appeals to you.

There are many hidden benefits from attending an exercise class, an important one being that it is a social diversion. You will be mixing with people of all shapes, ages and nationalities and even if you struggle with the routine to begin with, it will soon get easier. As well as being a healthy activity, you will find you have a load of new friends. Everybody is under so much stress today with so many worries and responsibilities that, I promise you, taking the time to get away from your daily life for an hour and joining a class with likeminded people will lift your spirits, help you eat more healthily and sleep more soundly than before. This is *your* time to do something good for yourself, to improve the shape of your body and quality of life.

Forget about focusing solely on diets; regular exercise is your key to maintaining a slim and healthy shape for the rest of your life. It doesn't have to be every day so that it becomes a drag. Aim for three times a week and put it in your diary so that you can arrange your daily schedule around your exercise time rather than vice versa. This will prevent the excuse of missing a session because of a meeting or appointment. But you have to find a form of exercise that you are prepared to do regularly. No one will stick at something they hate. There's no point in saying you are going to swim if you're not keen on getting wet, cold and a verruca. If, for you, the gym resembles a torture chamber and you don't fancy bouncing up and down on a mini trampoline, try something different like Zumba or table tennis. There are even classes for pole dancing. Who knew?!

So, what are you going to do? If you're still unconvinced take an honest look at your body shape, then check out the following:

EXERCISE CORRECTS YOUR POSTURE (DON'T LOSE YOUR NECK!)

Do you ever catch a glimpse of yourself in a mirror or shop window and think 'Who is that round-shouldered, grumpy-looking old person?' Quite a shock, isn't it? Next time you are in a cafe or restaurant, look at how people are sitting, particularly those who are obviously in their 60s or 70s. Many will be almost slumped over the table, their backs rounded, shoulders hunched. Where have their necks gone? (As you were reading that, did you instinctively sit up straighter and pull your shoulders back? Me too!) While habitual bad posture usually starts in our fifties, as a fitness instructor I am seeing it much earlier especially among people who use laptops or tablet computers.

The first stage is an almost imperceptible slump of the shoulders, mainly when you're tired at the end of a long day. This soon becomes your normal stance and causes your head to poke forward a little bit. You probably won't notice this happening as you soon get used to viewing the world around you from this angle. As time goes by though, the slump becomes more pronounced and your head pokes forward more until, when you're facing someone, it appears as if your neck has disappeared and your face is coming out of your chest! This posture also causes your tummy to stick out making you look like a question mark from the side. Not a good look.

To compensate for this unnatural posture, the bone at the top of your spine thickens to support the weight of your head, forming the unattractive dowager's hump. Sometimes this condition is hereditary but in many cases is simply a result of bad posture. If this becomes your habitual stance and you don't do any exercise to keep your shoulders and back supple, eventually you become 'locked' in this position and that's when people start complaining about pain and stiffness across their shoulders.

The obvious solution is to be aware if this is starting to happen and not let it get to that state. Imagine someone has taken hold of the hair at the top of your head (not the crown) and is gently pulling your head upwards towards the ceiling. Grow tall, lengthen your neck and pull your shoulders back and down a bit – just slightly, don't exaggerate the movement. Go on, try. How does that feel? A bit unnatural? Maybe, but hey, look – check in the mirror! Look at the difference. You appear slimmer, your sticky-out tummy has disappeared, and you look ten years younger. Just by standing up straight.

To further improve your posture, try some simple stretches; lift your arms above your head and reach up towards the ceiling with alternate arms to stretch out your spine. Then lower your arms and circle your shoulders back a few times to get rid of any tension. Just those simple moves will make you feel so much better.

If you can get into the habit of standing tall this will soon become your natural stance. If you can persuade a handy grandchild to take a picture of you in this straighter pose to keep on your mobile phone as a reminder to yourself, even better.

EXERCISE STRENGTHENS YOUR BONES

Every year after age 35 you lose roughly 1% of your bone mass making your bones more fragile, as described in chapter two. This is why a fall can often lead to a fractured wrist or femur. It is vitally important to keep your bones as strong as possible and for this you need weight-bearing exercise like walking, jogging and dancing, or sports where you run around like tennis.

The way it works is by putting your bones under stress. This might seem counterproductive but it's just the opposite. The large muscle groups, say, in your arms and legs, are attached to your bones by tendons, which are thick bands of fascia. When you subject your bones to tension such as jogging, each jolt makes the tendons pull on the bones forcing more amino acids into the cells of the bones making them stronger. The worst thing you can do is to sit around for long periods of time as this is the cause of most back pain. When you stand, your weight is evenly distributed across all your joints so no part is under undue strain. When you sit, all your weight is on your butt so more pressure goes through your spine and up into your neck especially if you slump. Very few people sit correctly – upright in their chair with their back and head supported – which is why the large muscles in your butt (the glutes) aren't stimulated and become weak, leading to gait abnormalities and pain when you walk. It's so easy to prevent that simply by moving around more.

Although cycling and swimming are good for other aspects of fitness, they don't contribute to bone strength, you need to be on your feet to make this happen. Have you noticed how kids dance nowadays in a club or at a music concert? They don't. They just jump up and down on the spot in time to the music. Excellent! They are going to have really strong bones. If going clubbing is not your thing and there is a step class at your gym, do try this. It simply entails going up and down on a stationary step in front of you and is an excellent way to strengthen your bones. Even if you are already doing some form of exercise, check out the next bit as well:

THE FOLLOWING EXERCISE IS VERY IMPORTANT AND SHOULD BE DONE EVERY DAY. IT TAKE LESS THAN ONE MINUTE AND COULD PREVENT YOU FROM GETTING OSTEOPOROSIS!

If you suffer from a bad back or any other skeletal or medical problem, please ignore the following – or check with a physiotherapist first.

Introducing Hop Along with Auntie Lee: Stand on your right leg, lift your left foot off the floor and hop up and down 4 times. Quickly switch to your left leg and repeat 4 hops. This is one set. Start off with this. If you find it difficult, do it in the kitchen with your hands pressing on the work surface to take some of the strain. Once you have managed one set – 4 hops on each leg – try two sets – without holding on and without stopping in between. This may make you a bit puffy. Gradually work up to four sets, 4 hops on your right leg, switching to 4 hops on the left leg, repeated four times. This will be 32 hops in all and will take less than a minute – I've timed it. It's that simple. When you have mastered that, try building up to 8 hops on each leg instead of 4. This is harder and if you follow the above you will end up doing 64 hops in all, but this still takes less than one minute.

Do this every day. Less than a minute! OK? Make it a ritual while waiting for the kettle to boil. I promise you the extra strength and endurance this will provide for your bones way exceeds the small amount of time and effort it takes. And because it makes you a bit puffy you are also strengthening your heart and lungs and increasing the circulation round your whole body. A little thing like this could stop osteoporosis in its tracks or prevent a breakage if you do happen to fall.

This is massively important and is much easier to do if you have some music playing, such as Aretha Franklyn singing 'Think' or 'Respect' which are both the right tempo. Just do it, yeah? I'm hopping you will!

EXERCISE CORRECTS YOUR BALANCE

You should be able to:

- Put your socks/boots on while standing on one leg
- Walk downstairs quite easily without holding on to a bannister or rail
- Feel safe walking on a frosty pavement

As people get older, their sense of balance can deteriorate. How often do you hear about someone's elderly aunt or uncle taking a tumble in the street, slipping on wet leaves or tripping over a rucked carpet? Obviously, any fall can cause a loss of confidence and make you more vulnerable with a fear of falling.

I do understand this; it can happen so easily and unexpectedly. I emerged from the shower recently and the bathmat I stepped on skidded slightly. If I hadn't grabbed hold of the basin for support, I might have gone flying! Just this small incident has made me more aware of my movements and environment.

I'm not as bad as my friend Nancy, though, who is my 'matinee buddy'; we go and see musicals together and are about to see *Hamilton* for the third time. Like a lot of people Nancy feels very unsteady going down stairs. She gingerly and slowly descends, one step at a time, sideways like a crab, holding on to the handrail with both hands. This is all very well at home but not when you're holding up all the passengers during rush hour at Tottenham Court Road tube station. I pretend I don't know her!

All types of exercise will give you stamina, muscle definition and help you burn fat, but for balance you need moves that are specifically focused on helping you stay upright on an uneven surface such as Yoga classes or slow, controlled movements like in Tai Chi.

If you do feel a bit wobbly, check with your doctor about specific balancing classes that are held at some NHS hospitals and get a referral. The sort of moves you will be taught are like the following which you could practise at home. Try this: Start by standing up straight as described above and pulling in your tummy before shifting your weight on to one leg. Lift the other foot off the floor and balance on one leg without holding on for as long as you can – then change to the other leg. Try and count to ten and gradually increase till you get to 20 seconds easily.

Make this a ritual, just something you do while engaged in another activity, like speaking on the phone or during the TV adverts. Some experts suggest standing on one leg while you clean your teeth, but even I can't do that because the hand and head movements, not to mention leaning over the basin, can throw anyone off balance! Once you are confident about balancing on one leg, try walking by putting one foot directly in front of the other as if on a tightrope – just as an exercise. Put your right foot in front of the left one so the right heel is touching your left toes and your feet are in a straight line (harder than it sounds!), then move the left foot in front in the same way and keep moving forward like that. Hold your arms out for balance. I bet you find this difficult at first. Confession: even I do, and I incorporate balancing exercises in my classes. Try it.

EXERCISE WILL GIVE YOU STRENGTH:
(GET A GRIP, WOMAN!)

How strong are your arms? Do you need two hands to lift that heavy saucepan full of water and potatoes off the stove to strain it? Can you grip a jar or bottle and unscrew it, or do you have to use a gadget or, even worse, copy me and jam the lid in the door frame? How many trips do you need to carry in a family-sized shop from your car to your kitchen? Is it one bag in each hand or can you manage two or three?

From the age of about 30 onwards, it's not only your bones that start to weaken but your muscles as well. Your muscles are made up of fibres which shrink through lack of use. This can lead to an accumulation of fat in the upper arms and the dreaded 'bingo wings.' As we discussed earlier, you can't help the skin changing texture as you get older, with wrinkles in the inner crease of the elbow and lines down the front of the arm, but if the underlying muscles are a good shape your arms will look much better at whatever age.

The only way to achieve nice toned arms and stop your shoulders from drooping – coat hanger shoulders – is some light weight training. I don't mean the bulgy, muscly look that some ageing celebrities go for, but I think you'll agree that a slim, firm-shaped arm is certainly more attractive than a limp or flabby one. To achieve this, look on the schedule of your health centre for a beginner's total workout class where you use light hand weights to tone and sculpt your arms. If this brings an image to your mind of those hairy weightlifters covered in Mazola heaving up a bar with the equivalent in weight of a Honda on each end, dispel it immediately. You will start by holding a 1kg (2.2lbs) in each hand and performing some simple moves to tone your arms. You will not get bulgy muscles from doing this.

When you do exercises like weight training, what is happening is that you are causing tiny, indeed miniscule, tears in the muscle fibres. During the following twenty-four hours these tiny tears are filled with protein so increasing the *density* of your muscles making them toned without bulking up. The good news is the more muscle you have, the more you can eat without putting on weight as muscle is 'metabolically active' meaning it encourages your body to burn up the food you are eating instead of storing it as fat.

With practice you should soon see a marked improvement in the shape of your arms and you might even feel confident enough to wear short-sleeved dresses and tops whatever your age. You will also be able to lift a small-sized grandchild with no problem.

EXERCISE WILL MAKE YOU FLEXIBLE

Can you reach up to get the biscuit tin down from a high shelf? Can you nimbly climb up on a chair to change a light bulb? How about bending down to do up your shoelace, getting in and out of the car with ease, and getting up from a deep armchair without going 'Ooof!'?

No problem, you say? Well, can you get down on the floor and up again without using your hands? Ah, bit more tricky.

I can't stress how important it is to keep flexible as you get older. How many times have you asked a friend how they are and they say, 'Well, my back has been playing up again.' In many cases this could be avoided by simple stretching exercises that help you to move your joints freely and keep your spine supple. The best classes for flexibility are Yoga, Pilates or a stretch and tone class. Any class that involves bending, twisting, stretching and lengthening your arms and legs will make you supple and prevent your spine from seizing up by strengthening the muscles in your back. Classes like Zumba or dance aerobics are excellent for flexibility as they use every muscle in the body.

These sorts of moves are also essential for preventing arthritis as they encourage the production of synovial fluid in your joints which lubricates them and stops the bones rubbing against each other which causes the pain of arthritis.

I've mentioned Yoga, above, but personally I am a bit ambivalent about it being a safe and beneficial form of exercise. Yoga has remained unchanged for hundreds of years and therefore has not kept up to date with the advances made by sports scientists. In my opinion certain poses where you take your legs higher than your head as in shoulder- and headstands and the 'plough' can be 'contra-indicated' for a beginner or older person. They put the neck in a vulnerable position as the whole of your body weight is resting on the delicate nerves and vertebrae at the top of your spinal column, and could cause lasting damage. *These moves should definitely not be attempted by anyone with glaucoma which many older people suffer from, as the pressure in your eyes can't adjust to the inverted position.*

Having said that, as the millions of Yoga devotees will attest, taught properly by a professional instructor, Yoga will make you strong and supple, improve balance and posture and induce a calmness of mind which will permeate into your daily life. So please don't let me put you off if this is something you'd like to try.

The bottom line is, keeping your shoulders, back and hips supple as you age is one of the best things you can do for your overall health. It will help you stay pain-free and hopefully you won't be joining your less mobile friends for a hip replacement any time soon.

EXERCISE WILL GIVE YOU STAMINA

Can you walk briskly up a hill without stopping halfway to catch your breath? How about running for a bus or climbing up three flights of stairs with ease? Lots of people have told me they didn't realise how unfit they've become until something happens that makes them compare their own fitness levels with the younger members of their family. For example, taking young grandchildren for a walk and trying to keep up with them as they run ahead. Then you wonder, how did that happen?

'I used to be so fit', they moan. 'I used to play tennis, drive into the countryside and go for long walks, go dancing – and never stopped to think I couldn't do this!'

So why don't you do that today? There is always an excuse or reason: an illness or injury, the loss of a partner with whom they used to share these activities, stress – or just a general lack of energy or loss of enthusiasm. It becomes easier not to bother and to seek more sedentary activities such as playing cards or Scrabble, meeting friends for lunch or watching daytime television.

Your body, however, was made to move! As I said earlier, if you don't make the effort, your muscles will grow weaker and lose the ability to support your joints adequately. That is why so many older people complain of aches and pains and stiffness, which contributes to feeling generally tired and listless. The obvious answer is to get up and move. On the days you don't go to a class, make the commitment to go for a walk, come rain or shine. Map out a route for yourself, walk around the block – choose a distance of about a mile that takes 15 to 20 minutes to cover – and if this incorporates a slight slope or even a hill – all the better.

However busy you are, you must be able to find a twenty-minute slot sometime in your day. Don't aim for longer as that just lets in the excuse that you 'don't have time.' If you haven't got a pair of training shoes already, buy yourself a good, comfortable pair made by a recognised brand. They may be expensive, but this is your passport to health. Be advised by the expert in the sports shop.

Each night, lay out the clothes you are going to wear for your walk the next day, with your trainers ready where you can see them. Try and fit this walk in first thing in the morning before your mind can register objections about all the things you're planning to do for the rest of the day. Those emails can wait, so can the phone calls. When you walk, be aware of lifting your feet and taking big strides with a confident heel-toe action through each foot, swinging your arms as you go. If you want to do this with a friend, there are advantages and disadvantages. The positive aspect is making the commitment so you would feel guilty for letting your friend down if you woke up one morning with a 'can't be bothered' attitude. The negative side is if *she* lets *you* down because she is waiting for the washing machine man / an Amazon or Ocado delivery / her cleaner – and so on. However, if your friend is as keen as you are, then go for it – make it a ritual!

Whether you set out alone or phone a friend, once this daily walk is ingrained into your psyche, you will feel irritated if anything happens that causes you to miss it one day. After a few weeks you will have increased your stamina to such as extent you'll be hearing 'Hey, Grandma, wait for us!'

LOOKING GOOD (DON'T LOSE YOUR SHAPE)

When you look at photos of yourself as a teenager or young woman, don't you think how lovely you were then and how little you appreciated that at the time? A firm body, slim, toned legs, a neat waist (where's that gone now?) and a round bottom that filled out your trousers or shorts nicely.

And now – you don't even want think about it let alone examine your naked body in the mirror! As you approach your seventh or eighth decade there is nothing you can do about loss of height or skin elasticity. It just can't be helped. However, it's never too late to start taking some simple steps to improve your overall shape – beginning with 'Don't get fat.' Now she tells us! Come on now, fat is ageing and just increases your inclination to shun all forms of movement.

As well as that daily walk to increase your stamina, you also need some simple exercises to tone your tummy muscles and lift and tone your bottom which will make an enormous difference to the way you look and your energy levels. In particular, you need to work on your core muscles, the band of muscle in your lower torso that supports your internal organs. Rather than describe any specific exercises here, I would encourage you to attend an exercise class so that a professional fitness instructor can show you how to do these properly. A beginner's body conditioning class is a good start and is often listed on the timetable as 55+ so don't be afraid to try this even if you are in your 70s or 80s.

Although it is my job to encourage people to take regular exercise if they want to be slim, toned and healthy I've found that, generally, amongst my peers, there is a marked reluctance to heed my advice. People would rather control their weight by dieting than burn up the calories through exercise. Do you recognise any of the excuses below?

'I HAVEN'T GOT TIME!'

I notice you manage to find time to get your nails manicured, and I'm sure you haven't missed an episode of your favourite weekly TV programme for years! You *do* have time. If you had to go to the dentist you would put the appointment in your diary. So surely, if you really wanted, you could find three spare half-hours to do something, even if it's dancing around the kitchen to your favourite music– or imitating your teenage grandchildren by jumping up and down.

'I'M TOO FAT/OLD TO START NOW'

No, you're not. If you can put one foot in front of the other, you're not too fat to walk on a treadmill for ten minutes, and as for being too old, there's no such thing – unless you are incapacitated in some way. Find one of those council-run 55+ classes which are very inexpensive and just the thing to get you started.

What about trying a class with a friend, just for a laugh? You can't become fit if you've never seen other old people *being* fit, and you will be surprised at how many older people, of all shapes and sizes, there are in the class. Go on, try. You'll be amazed at the difference it will make to your general health when you get a bit fitter.

'I'M EXHAUSTED AFTER HAVING THE GRANDCHILDREN. IT TAKES ME A DAY TO RECOVER'

I understand that, but however tired you may be, a different environment with music and cheerful people soon changes your mood, and if you can find a nice dance class with funky music from your era, you would soon find yourself up and dancing with the rest of them.

'I DON'T WANT TO GET ALL HOT AND SWEATY – MY HAIR WILL GO FRIZZY.'

Oh well, we can't have that now, can we! Actually, the older you are, the less you will sweat – fact. Well to be precise, you sweat differently, particularly if you are a woman. This is related to the menopause – hot flushes – but researchers have found that sweat glands, especially under the arms, shrink and become less sensitive as you age, which translates into reduced perspiration production. So that knocks that one on the head!

'IT'S SO BORING'

Your muscles will only get toned by doing the same movement over and over again, so I agree, by dint of repetition, exercise can be boring. But, so is cleaning your teeth and removing your makeup but you wouldn't neglect those, would you? Exercise needn't be boring if you're prepared to try different things: what about taking some tennis lessons or ballroom dancing? Kickboxing is fun – I did that for two years and punching pads held by a trainer is great for releasing tension. I visualised the face of someone who cheated my husband in business and got a lot of satisfaction when I jabbed and hooked! Perhaps the opposite of that, if you enjoyed dancing as a child, are ballet barre classes which will improve your posture and give you a great body.

'WON'T EXERCISE SIMPLY STIMULATE MY APPETITE AND MAKE ME EVEN MORE HUNGRY?'

No – just the opposite actually. Continuous movement stimulates the liver to release stored glucose. When this increased level of glucose is perceived by the hypothalamus – the part of your brain that controls hunger – it correctly assumes that you don't need food right now, so the hunger signals are not activated.

'I'VE GOT A BAD BACK' / 'I'VE GOT A BAD BACK' / 'I'VE GOT A BAD BACK'

That's because you don't exercise! Seriously, if you do have problems with your spine or surrounding muscles, do check with an osteopath or physiotherapist and see what they say. My guess is that they will reinforce the old adage; if you don't use it, you lose it, and advise you to keep moving as much as possible.

Fact: people who exercise regularly give the impression of being much younger than they are; that comes from being slim, able to move easily, and having lots of energy. Fact: people who don't exercise appear bulky and shapeless, move stiffly and look much older than their years. The point is, you need to change your body from fat-storing to fat-burning. This is done by raising your metabolic rate – which is the rate at which your body uses food for energy – through exercise and eating the right kind of food. As I explained in the last chapter, sugary food gets stored as fat. Protein such as chicken, fish and eggs, combined with vegetables and fruit get burned up as energy.

Everyone, and I mean *everyone*, who has lost excess weight and kept it off has incorporated a regular session of exercise into their life. It doesn't matter what it is but the action of getting into your fitness 'uniform' – trainers, tracksuit, swimsuit or lycra workout gear – promotes a feeling of 'body awareness' and the fact that you are about to do something beneficial for your body and your general health. After a satisfying workout, you wouldn't want to go home and eat junk food; this would just negate everything you've just done. Exercise makes you more aware of your body and fosters a desire to take better care of it.

I hope I've convinced you. If so, what are you prepared to do on a regular basis? Here are some suggestions for various types of exercise you could do:

SWIMMING

You burn calories and build muscle while swimming because of the resistance of the water. As your muscles are pushed harder, so your heart and lungs have to increase their capacity to pump oxygen around your body which improves your cardiovascular health. This is also good if you have arthritis as the water supports 90% of your body weight causing less painful movements in the affected joints. Try an 'aqua aerobic' class and see how you get on.

My friend Linda: 'You have to get wet, cold, frizzy hair, damp towels, gender neutral changing rooms...'

OK then, what about ...

CYCLING

Riding a bike burns more calories than jogging with less impact on your joints, especially your knees, as sitting in the saddle takes the strain. You get lots of fresh air if you cycle outdoors, especially in the countryside. If you prefer to remain indoors you have the compensation of a TV screen in front of you in a gym to take your mind of the fact that you are working pretty hard!

My friend Nancy: 'Sitting on the hard saddle for ages gave me thrush.'

Me: 'It did not!'

GOLF

Lots of women take this up once they retire. It's pretty good exercise as you're stretching and twisting to hit the ball which improves your flexibility, balance and core strength. As golf courses are not flat, you'll burn lots of calories walking up and down hilly terrain. My friend Adie took up golf in her 70s and is able to hit the ball a huge distance – sadly not in the direction of the hole, but I guess that will come in time. Taking a buggy defeats the purpose!

My friend Nancy: 'I went with Adie and thought the women at her posh golf club were cliquey and unfriendly.'

Oh.

WALKING FOOTBALL

Who would have thought?! This has really taken off since it was created in 2011. There are men's and women's teams all over the country especially for the over 50s. The rules mean no running, just walking up to the ball and kicking it. If you run, the other side gets a free kick. What a great way to keep your legs moving without overdoing it – and giving your grandchildren a laugh!

My friend Dilly: 'Don't be ridiculous!'

NORDIC WALKING

Normal everyday walking gets the blood pumping round the body without putting too much strain on your cardio-vascular system and also revs up your metabolic rate to burn fat. Nordic walking is one step up from this. Holding a pole in each hand and propelling yourself along through the city or countryside burns up 46% more calories than ordinary walking. It's rather like skiing without the snow. As Nancy Sinatra didn't sing: 'these poles were made for walking.' There are groups around the country to help you get to grips (ha ha) with this.

My friend Adele: 'And you look like a total prat!'

BEING FIT PROTECTS YOUR BRAIN

There is another, serious reason why you, as a not-so-young person, need to be physically strong and that is to protect a very important part of your anatomy – your brain. As well as the benefits described above, being fit can prevent a serious condition that sometimes develops in older people immediately after having an operation under a general anaesthetic, which is why I have included it in the chapter on exercise. It is known in the medical profession as post-operative cognitive decline (POCD), the symptoms being mild to moderate memory loss and behaviour changes; somehow your responses are just not as sharp as before. Worryingly, this can sometimes last for weeks and in some extreme cases may also increase the risk of dementia, the theory being that the general anaesthesia may contribute to brain inflammation and thus encourage the production of amyloid plaques, which are linked to Alzheimer's disease. Bit scary, that!

Obviously not everyone suffers from post-operative cognitive decline but the longer the surgery and the older – *and more unfit* – you are, the higher the risk of developing the condition. Don't blame me, I'm merely the messenger!

The answer, obviously, is to try and avoid having a general anaesthetic. As my husband's doctor said to me after his quadruple heart bypass: 'Get him home as soon as possible. Hospital is no place for sick people – too many germs!'

If you are scheduled to have an operation in the near future, your surgeon will encourage you to get as fit as possible prior to going into hospital. Exercise, especially that which makes you a bit puffy, like fast walking or dancing, will increase blood and oxygen supply to your brain which will ensure a better outcome and faster recovery time. And you won't go loopy afterwards!

Look after your brain and your body. Only you can make the commitment to do this. You only have one life so why not live the rest of it as a slim and healthy person. The time is now.

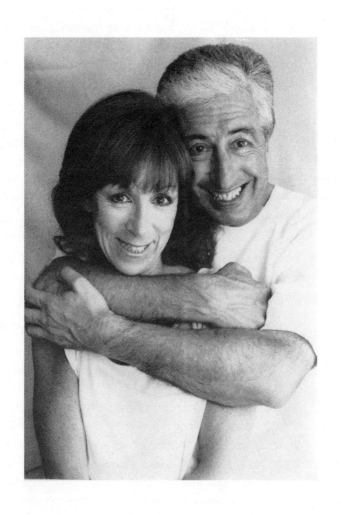

9

GRIEF IS LOVE UNWILLING TO LET GO

The tone of this book has been deliberately flippant because, as actress Bette Davis said: 'Old age ain't for cissies.' However, there is one subject where no amount of frivolity can be justified: that of grief, the loss of someone you love. Unfortunately, nearly everyone who survives into their 70s and 80s will have experienced the death of a close relative or friend.

Therefore, I cannot write a book about getting older without touching on this subject. I did hesitate though, in case I came across as being self-indulgent, or writing an exercise in personal catharsis but, in spite of all the books and articles written about losing a loved one and the proliferation of counselling services, nothing prepares you for the actual experience when it happens.

Just as all the information and classes you can attend are supposed to prepare you for childbirth, the actual event is completely individual and nothing like you've been told to expect. It is the same with losing someone close, because however many funerals you go to of friends and, hopefully elderly, relatives, nothing hits you like the death of your husband or wife especially if you have been married for a great many years.

DEATH HAPPENS

My beloved husband, Maurice Djanogly OBE, was diagnosed with stomach cancer in May 2014 and died aged 81 on 8 December that same year.

A charming, highly intelligent, articulate man he was equally at home socialising with his friends in the House of Lords as he was surrounded by grandchildren, chatting to the waitress in Nando's.

I loved him with all my heart. I know it's a cliché, but he was my rock. In fact I only ventured out to try things by myself – like setting up and running my own fitness studio, *All That Jazz*, in the 80s, or sending manuscripts to publishers in the 90s with the usual expectation of adding to my collection of rejection slips – so I could scurry back to the protection of his arms. Nothing mattered so long as he was there.

Why am I telling you this? Because no one really wants to talk about the feelings and day-to-day experiences of the bereaved. You have heard of people crossing the street pretending not to see you because they just don't know what to say. I can understand that.

I must have sounded crass on occasions when I intended to be sympathetic, because, well, what did I know?

So, I decided I *would* talk about the immediate and continuing aftermath of losing my husband with other women of my age and see what comes up. Well, I can tell you, there are a lot of us 'widder women' out there! (sorry guys, there weren't many of you in our discussions). I know it's a rather unconventional response to 'how are you?' by saying 'I'm a bit down because my husband died and I just found a half finished crossword under the bed and couldn't stop crying.' This would elicit a response such as 'Oh I know what you mean because ...' or 'I never told this to anyone before but...'

The genuine relief that other people felt the same and we were all in the same boat was palpable. Just talking to an ordinary person who has been through a similar experience and is not a professional counsellor has made a big difference for them, and for me. So, if you have suffered a similar loss and this chapter helps you, then I'm really pleased.

There were a lot of similarities in the attitudes of the women I spoke to, such as: 'no one wants to be with someone who is miserable so you have to try and put on a cheerful face'; 'I don't want to bore people with my sorrows'; 'I feel that the children are "watching" me and willing me to behave normally so they can go home and not feel guilty that I am alone.' I confessed to two women at an exercise class I attend that, even after five years, I still have my husband's favourite fleecy jacket on my bed as he really felt the cold and wore it every day. I give it a hug every morning and tell him my plans for the day. One of the other women whose husband died two years ago said her husband's pyjamas are still under the pillow next to hers; the other one admitted she had to get her children to pack up her deceased husband's clothes – as did I – because she couldn't face doing it, but still kept his ties hanging in the cupboard.

After some of the chats I would get emails along the lines of: 'I can't thank you enough for lifting my spirits like you did. I got more out of our talk than three months of counselling and felt so much better. I now realise I'm not the only one who thought she was going mad!'

No, you're not going mad. We all felt like that sometimes.

Another lady wrote, 'I lost my husband six years ago and the people around me assume I have "got over it by now". They even suggest it would be nice if I "met someone else". Well I haven't got over it and it was such a relief to admit that and to realise that other women felt the same. Counselling helped me during the sessions, but then I went home to an empty house and cried.'

There are many phrases in common parlance to describe death, as if to make it a softer option, such as 'passed away' or simply, 'he's gone.' Personally, I dislike the expression 'I've lost my husband.' It smacks of carelessness; as though I have left him on the tube and expect him to turn up in the lost property office in Baker Street. I wish. I didn't 'lose' him. He died.

THE AFTERMATH

Most bereaved people do find solace in counselling. Many don't find it helpful. I guess it's such a personal thing and greatly dependent on whether you trust the counsellor enough to unburden yourself to him or her. Although I had lots of kindly offers from various organisations after my husband died, I didn't want to sit opposite someone with an 'understanding' look on their face and cry. Possibly I should have done because there were occasions when I just wanted to rant and scream about the unfairness of it, but I didn't in the end. The only thing I would want to know from a counsellor is whether they could bring my husband back to me. If not, then I'm not interested.

Maybe Dr Elizabeth Kubler Ross had something when she described the framework for learning to live with the grief of loss: denial, anger, bargaining, depression and finally, acceptance. These are tools to help identify what we may be feeling. Maybe they are, but I found these are not stations on some linear timeline of grief. They don't happen in that order and some won't come up at all. For example, if your husband or loved one is terminally ill and you have to go through all the horrors of their decline, in the end you are praying for them to die and put an end to their suffering. So, when it happens, your first feeling is one of relief for them – then guilt that you feel that way.

According to Dr Kubler Ross:

Denial is pretending it hasn't happened: he's just gone to pay the paper bill, be back soon.

(Please come back soon.)

Rather than denial is disbelief: I can't believe he isn't here anymore. Panic: I don't know where he is. Anguish: I don't know how to *be* without him. Then the tears. Not just the tears but when you're alone, the howling – loud, uncontrollable howling, keening, rocking back and forth. When that pain strikes, it's real, it's physical, you are doubled up as though someone has stuck a knife into you. A part of you is outside yourself watching, bewildered: 'Who are you? Why are you making that noise? I've never seen you like that. Stop it, the neighbours will hear.' It can last for up to an hour then finally you subside, exhausted.

If anyone tells you crying is a good thing and you'll feel better afterwards, they are totally wrong. That sort of crying just leaves you with a red nose, puffy eyes and a blinding headache. Maybe psychologically it's 'good to let it all out', but it's extremely painful, I can tell you.

I realised those extreme bouts of crying were a release from having to remain calm and outwardly cheerful by the bedside of my dying husband. Mo – as he was affectionately known – would say 'I don't want to leave you' and start to cry. I would say, 'I'll be all right, why do you think we had five children?' and he would smile and relax. Then I would drive home almost blinded by tears so I could barely see where I was going.

Anger: no, I'm not angry with my husband – he truly wanted to stay with us. My friend Judy was furious with her husband who died suddenly on the way back from a party. Luckily, she was driving so when he complained of chest pain, she drove straight to the A&E of her local hospital. He died a few hours later and she was cross with him for ages afterwards because he left her without warning. 'I was sitting in the waiting room wearing my party dress and my Jimmy Choos,' she said irrationally.

The only anger I felt was towards the practice of oncology, although not the man who treated my husband; he was kind and came through for us in the end. It's the work ethic many adopt. All I can say is God protect us from over-zealous oncologists who seem to think that dying is failure. Of course, not all of them are like that, and this is obviously a personal opinion but I feel that too many oncologists offer false hope which, as scared, newly diagnosed patients, we clutch at, willing to do anything to stay with the people we love and who love us.

The oncologist will argue that all the treatments are fully explained to the patient and they have a choice whether to go ahead with the treatment. But do they? Really? When you are desperately ill and sitting opposite an all-powerful doctor who holds your life in his hands and who says 'you have six months to live but with chemotherapy we may be able to shrink the tumour and give you another two years, tops.' Is that really a choice? Look, I get it – really, I do. Doctors want to be seen to be doing something – taking action. To advise doing nothing feels like giving in and being unsupportive towards the patient. But is the 'something' always in the best interest of the patient, putting them through hell for what – a few extra months of life?

I don't mean to sound totally negative. Naturally every case is different, and most of the time chemotherapy is warranted and successful in buying valuable time for the patient. We all have friends who have been through the horror of breast cancer and come out the other side, cured. The doctors can only use the tools at their disposal and I firmly believe they do the best they can. But it's easier for them to do what they know best, what their core training is geared towards – which is to continue treatment in pursuit of a cure.

I'm not going into details about my husband's treatment, although you would have an idea from what I've written here. Chemotherapy is a barbaric treatment with horrendous side effects and as his gastroenterologist said to me after his death, 'With hindsight I wish I hadn't pointed him towards an oncologist.' You think?! I have to state, though, that the London hospital he was in could not have cared for him more tenderly and lovingly right up until the end.

My younger son thinks in fifty years we will look back on chemotherapy and radiotherapy as primitive as the way we now think of blood-sucking leeches as a cure for ailments. New preventative treatments in the form of immunotherapy are being developed all the time and have been highly successful in revving up the immune system to eliminate tumours in certain cancers. Hopefully non-invasive cures for cancer will be available on the NHS for everyone eventually.

For my husband, losing his hair was a big deal. He was not in any way a vain man but he had lovely thick grey hair which he kept neatly trimmed and immaculate. I'm sure for women it must be a lot worse but wigs today are very realistic and many of my friends unfortunate enough to develop cancer still felt feminine and happy to socialise wearing a good quality wig. For men like Mo it can make them feel diminished. I know he hated seeing himself that way. I bought him a navy beanie hat which he wore all the time, mainly because of the cold. The last photo I have of him a couple of days before he died is a selfie, surrounded by three of his adult children, all four of them wearing beanie hats in support and laughing into the camera.

The BBC television series *Horizon* aired a programme called 'We need to talk about death' on 23 January 2019. The discussion was about when is the right time to stop aggressive medical treatments. I wrote down the following quote word-for-word from the wonderful Professor Rob George, medical director of St Christopher's Hospice in south London, who said: 'I think it's morally wrong to waste a dying person's time and one of the easiest ways to waste a dying person's time is to offer them treatments which you know jolly well are going to make very little difference.'

Professor George is of the opinion that palliative care in a hospice should be considered much earlier once a patient is diagnosed with advanced cancer. As he said, 'Managing pain is not that difficult. The emphasis in a hospice is on the life that is left, the life that somebody is leaving, the life they are completing. There is a choice to say maybe I should just enjoy the time that's left and do the things that make me human rather than make my blood test better. Hospices are places for the living to get the best quality of life until they die. Palliative care is about improving people's symptoms: controlling things like pain, nausea, vomiting, breathlessness. It is about improving the situation of a patient faced with the most frightening prospect – the knowledge that he or she is going to die.'

Twenty years ago, a hospice was associated solely with death and dying and considered to be the last stop on the Life Line terminating at Cemetery. Palliative care was tacked on to the end of life when all hope was gone. Most people still believe that, myself included, until I saw that programme. How wrong we are. Now people living with cancer can be admitted for days at a time to be given the necessary drugs to control their symptoms then return to their families to live as normal a life as possible. For some people this can go on for years allowing them to do what's important to them and having the energy to do so.

I firmly believe that people should be given more informa-tion and more choice in whether to accept treatment *with all that entails* or opt for palliative care – although this may mean that they die sooner. The decision is whether it's worth it if there is a certain percentage of success. Interestingly, the doctor presenting the programme took a survey of many of his medical colleagues and they *all* said they would not choose prolonged treatment unless the result would guar-antee them the same standard of life they had before.

How early in the stage of the disease palliative care is opted for has to be decided between patient and doctor. It's not either/or but an extra layer of support. I know what I would have wanted for my husband. I just wish I'd had more knowledge at the time. Instead of my darling man spending his last few weeks languishing in a hospital bed being treated for the side effects of, supposedly, 'gentle' chemotherapy, he could have been pottering along to his club to play cards and darts with his friends, sitting in the garden in the sunshine doing the *Times* crossword and hugging his beloved grandchildren.

So no, I'm not angry, I only want to pass on to you, my reader, what I have learned and if it helps you to make an informed decision in the future, I'm glad. I just wish I'd known there was a choice. Now you do.

The **bargaining** stage can go on for a while: I would give anything – five years of my life – to have him back just for one day in good health. 'Please, just come back, I will never ask you to take the bins out ever again, I promise.'

As for **depression** it's difficult to differentiate whether you are really depressed or just inordinately, deeply sad. You try to put on a cheerful face for the children but your heart aches for them. After all they have also lost their daddy whom they loved more than anything in the world. I know some women find that a short course of antidepressants or sleeping pills does see them through the first difficult weeks, but there is always the tendency to revert back to the pills for future upsets instead of facing and dealing with them.

SUPPORT SYSTEMS

If you have been through this sort of bereavement, I hope you had the amount of support that I did. Not only my children who were amazing, taking it in turns to leave their families and stay with me for the odd night, but friends who popped in with food and stayed for a chat. But not everyone gets it right. Some of the things people say are intended to be helpful but often have the opposite effect. Don't say things like:

'At least he lived a long life.' Not long enough for me.

"He's in a better place.' No, he isn't. His place is next to me at the kitchen table.

'I know how you feel.' No, you don't.

'Time is a great healer.' Maybe eventually, but not at this moment.

'You'll find someone else.' I don't want anyone else, I just want him.

And please don't do 'the look.' You know the one: head on one side, face contorted in a grimace of exaggerated concern as if to say, 'I am sharing your pain.' I know you mean well but I'm trying to hold it together here and you are not helping. Please don't do this, it feels totally false and irritates rather than comforts.

It's best to keep it simple. Good things to say:

'I am so sorry.'

'I'm thinking of you and sending love and strength to get through this.'

'My favourite memory of him is …'

'I'm only a phone call away – any time you want to talk – I mean it.'

'I go to Tesco every tuesday so let me know if you need anything.'

'I wish I could make it better.'

'He told everyone how much he loved you.'

'I've brought you the perfect mango.'

A brief hug and a murmured 'This is shit, isn't it?' to which you can reply 'Yeah' is a better greeting than forced jollity which feels unnatural. Those are good friends.

As well as fantastic children, what everyone really needs at a time like this is a sister. My sister, Marilyn (her real name!), is my support and soulmate and we speak on the phone morning and evening. We couldn't be more different in looks (she is beautiful), tastes (I like lemon curd and eat it out the jar with a teaspoon, she grimaces with disgust), clothes (she is smart, elegant, designer-savvy whereas I am – not!) and interests (she absolutely loves her car, I don't even know the make of mine!). What we do share, however, is a sense of humour. I can be quite funny (can't I?) but when we are together something will start us off and we are soon doubled up with laughter. Yet try to explain to a third party what is so funny, and they won't get it. I guess it's a sister thing. After all who else can you rely on for everything from dealing with elderly parents to a crisis such as this? She would turn up at the hospital and say, 'I'll stay with him for a while, why not take a break and go for a walk in the sunshine.' Even in the depths of my despair she could still make me laugh. Hours before Mo died, I phoned her from the hospital corridor and sobbed, 'He's so bad, I can't do this anymore.' She said, 'Don't move, I'm coming,' and was there in minutes still with a clip in her hair.

You also need help with the dreaded probate. This is the legal and financial process involved in dealing with property, money and possessions – that is, the assets – of the dead person. It can be a convoluted nightmare encompassing lots of complicated legal, tax and financial work, which requires the assistance of a friendly and helpful solicitor to sort it all out. It can be costly and time-consuming, but the terms of the will can't be carried out until this is completed.

If ever you have to go through – or have gone through – the experience of probate, I hope you were as lucky as I was to have a financially savvy son-in-law like Steve, who willingly took on the task of sorting out my husband's tangled myriad of financial affairs. It took him several months of painstakingly visiting banks, building societies, writing endless letters and, finally, getting probate granted. Steve's advice would be to pay for about 15 copies of the death certificate – expensive but necessary – as every organisation you deal with requests an original, properly authorised certificate, and you can't keep sending the original one out then demanding it back.

The case of his favourite wine that I present him with every now and again is barely adequate for the years he has spent taking my anguished phone calls: 'My computer has died,' 'I've had this strange email', 'someone's bashed into my car.' He manages my energy suppliers – changing companies when necessary – sorts my financial affairs and does my yearly tax return.

I hope you have a Steve – and a daughter like the one who wisely chose to marry him.

AND AFTER THAT

The silence. The house is so quiet. The children have gone home, having been persuaded to go back to their families with the reassurance that I'll be fine. You are alone. Sure, you've been alone in the house for several hours before, but this is a different sort of quiet – it's, well, a 'something missing' quiet. If you do inadvertently say something out loud, you are startled by the sound of your own voice.

When you've been married for a long time, love mellows into a rock solid friendship and unity. You can tell when a couple has that oneness when you see them catch each other's eye in a crowded room, such as at a party, and one will give a little secret signal which the other instantly understands, and they share a conspiratorial smile. We had that.

Other people did too. A woman I really admire is Dame Esther Rantzen. Who would have thought of initiating a telephone counselling service like *Childline* for troubled children to turn to for help and advice? And not only think of it but do all the slog to get it up and running – brilliant! Dame Esther seemed to have had the same loving relationship with her husband, the television producer Desmond Wilcox, as I had with Maurice. She was desperately lonely after his premature death in 2000 which she aptly described as, 'having plenty of people to do something with but nobody to do nothing with.' Isn't that just the perfect description?

Dame Esther is also the founder/president of a similar set-up for older people called The Silver Line which is 'committed to improving the lives of older people who are affected by loneliness and isolation.' So, anyone who is feeling a bit down and just wants to chat to a friendly person can call 0800 4 70 80 90 at any time, day or night. How enterprising it that!

The dancer, Debbie McGee, also had that special relationship with her husband, Paul Daniels. In an interview she said she is convinced that the grief she suffered after his death caused her breast cancer. Saying she felt lost going through the 'harrowing' battle without him, she added, 'I've never been through the stress I've been through since I lost Paul. Grief hits you in so many ways you're not expecting. It's not all about sadness.' Luckily Debbie's tumours were discovered early through her regular screening and were removed.

I'm sure many of us can identify with both these women. Fame and recognition don't protect you from the realities of life.

NOW WHAT?

Who will help me fold the sheets when they come out of the tumble dryer? Who will zip up my dress before I go out? Who will watch as I climb up on a chair to change a light bulb in case I fall? Who will say, 'It's probably nothing' and 'Don't let it get to you, you know what she's like' and 'how about a nice cup of tea?'

The first thing I did after the funeral was to change to another doctor's surgery. I had been wanting to do that for years because of the shambolic administration and utter rudeness of the three receptionists in the present one, but Mo really liked the head of the practice who seemed to have time for him, so I put up with it. I reckoned I had no reason to do so any longer so applied to another surgery. Filling in the form gave me my first jolt: it asked for marital status. I had to put 'widow.' Widow! I am a widow! What a horrible word. I choked up.

Next hurdle: my daughter's birthday card. I couldn't, absolutely *could not* just sign it with the single word

'Mum.' In the end I put, 'With all our love, Mum-on-earth and Dad-in-heaven.' More tears – from both of us.

It's the little unexpected things that throw you: seeing an elderly couple, the man with grey hair just like Mo's, walking hand in hand through Marks & Spencer. Blinking back tears makes your throat close up and you have difficulty swallowing. What you want to avoid in public is some kindly soul enquiring anxiously, 'Are you all right?' You can only force a smile and nod.

Going out with friends for a meal is tricky when you are the only one without a partner. The usual combination is two or three couples together and at the end of the meal, when presented with the bill, the men normally all put their credit cards on the saucer and leave the waiter to divide it by three. The first time you are invited out with your regular friends, the other two couples will insist on paying for you. Let them, it's fine. After that, I suggest you keep some ten-pound notes in your bag and when the bill comes, depending on how high-end a restaurant you are at, put the requisite number of notes on the table as your contribution to the meal. Your friends will protest at first, but say, very firmly, 'Please let me do this.' They will sense how important this is to you and reluctantly agree.

What about when you are invited to parties and weddings? Are you happy to go on your own? Even after all this time, I can't say I am. If it's a family affair, obviously one of my children will take me and ensure I'm not left alone. I can't do wedding parties, however. If it's the son or daughter of a friend, I'm quite happy to go to the religious service, but I explain to my friends beforehand that I won't be coming to the reception and dinner-dance. They will understand and, if they don't, too bad!

Three weeks after Mo died, it was Christmas. These holidays, like birthdays and New Year celebrations, are very hard to deal with. All my family come for lunch at my house on Christmas Day and we have turkey and chestnut stuffing, the whole works. Five children, their partners, seven grandchildren and my sister and her husband are a lot of people to fit round the table, but we manage. What should I do about the empty place at the head of the table this year? I solved this by putting my two teenage grandsons in Mo's place and we drank a toast to him and the full and productive life he led.

His birthday was another milestone to be overcome. We all went to the cemetery with my youngest granddaughter, then aged 7, who brought three balloons already inflated with helium. Everyone wrote a happy birthday message on the balloons and we let them go and watched as they drifted up to heaven where the youngster was sure her beloved grandpa would read them.

You can't avoid the extra feelings of grief at these times and family support is invaluable. My sister knew, instinctively, when I was feeling desolate and weepy. The doorbell would ring and she would be standing there saying, 'I was just passing so I thought I would drop in.' What, at 8.00 in the morning? 5.30 in the evening? I don't think so! But it was so lovely to see her, and she would get me through the next hour and not leave until I was calm and able to cope again. Everyone needs someone intuitive like that, be it a family member or close friend.

The weeks go by and you think you're doing fine; your spirits have lifted a little, you are able to look at family photos, laugh at silly television programmes and people have stopped giving you 'the look.' But then you catch sight of his favourite biscuits that you don't buy anymore in the supermarket, and the loss sweeps over you again like a wave. You desperately want to feel his arms around you in a hug. You want him to be at home when you get there to help bring the shopping in from the car. You want to hear him say, 'What are we watching tonight?' as he scans the TV pages. The realisation that none of that is going to happen is like a blow to your heart. My only consolation was reminding myself that I was going through this hell so he wouldn't have to. Maybe that is a sentiment that would help you too if you ever needed it? I could not imagine Maurice coping on his own if I had died first. He had an indulgent mother who did everything for him, and I just took over once we married – willingly. That's just how it was in those days.

On the plus side: you no longer have to iron shirts, ('I'd gladly do this if only ...' that *bargaining* stage revisited), you have sole control of the TV remote, you can cancel the Sky Sports Channel and save a bit of money, the dishwasher only goes on once a week, if that – it's only one plate so you just wash that up – and you don't have to be nice to the wife of his friend from the golf club, who made it plain she didn't like you because you're slim and she's fat.

ACCEPTANCE

We need to talk about death. It allows us to prepare, it helps us to grieve and it leads us to an acceptance of what is inevitable for all of us. Only an acceptance of death can empower us with choice, allow us to stay in control and reclaim the narrative of our lives right to the end, to die a better death ourselves.

I read somewhere that it takes two years and four months to feel 'normal' after a traumatic event like the loss of a partner. In the depths of grief, you don't believe you will ever feel normal again and wish people would stop saying 'Give it time, you'll see.' They are right – partly. In my case, it took two years and *five* months when I woke up one morning and suddenly realised I hadn't cried for two days. It wasn't that I had stopped thinking about Mo, but I could do so without the black cloud of sadness descending upon me.

I was watching a television series called *Sensitive Skin* on Sky Arts, written by Hugo Blick and starring Kim Cattrall as the owner of an art gallery. At the end of series one, her husband died suddenly. This being a black comedy, in series two her dead husband kept popping up unexpectedly, offering advice when she was dealing with a client, which only she could hear. She would tell him to go away and stop interfering, leaving the client looking bewildered and wondering who she was talking to. He would pop up again when she was out on a date, sitting on a spare chair at the table much to her annoyance. In the end she confessed to her therapist (naturally) how irritating this was, and his advice was, 'You have to mentally and physically let him go. Actually say out loud "you have to go now, darling, goodbye," and it will stop happening.' She eventually did, after a lot of heart searching. I can't do that. I don't want to say goodbye to him. I like to feel Mo's presence in the house and imagine the white feathers I keep finding in odd places are messages from him. He certainly sent me a beautiful red butterfly a few weeks after his death. At the time I didn't realise butterflies are considered to be messengers from departed loved ones. Who knew? This one settled near my chair in the garden and closed and opened its wings as though trying to tell me something. I amused myself by copying the movement with my hands.

The following day I was sitting in the sunshine again when the same – I'm sure of it – butterfly flew over the hedge, seeming to make a beeline for me, and landed *on my arm*. I was too surprised to move. After a minute it flew up and over my head and landed *on my other arm*. It stayed there for a while then settled again by my chair. Eventually I got up to go inside and the butterfly went nuts; it flew round and round my chair then round my head then round the chair again before flying off over the hedge. It was a very weird experience. Was it trying to tell me to stay a while longer in the garden? Was it a message from Mo telling me he had arrived safely in heaven and was watching out for me? I wonder. I only know that the following year, a red butterfly actually flew in through the open window of my living room. It circled the room a couple of times while I watched, not knowing quite what to do, then settled on the curtain. I got a glass and managed to coax it inside before releasing it out of the window. Hi Mo, thank you for the visit.

The singer Gary Barlow and his wife suffered a terrible loss when their little daughter, Poppy, was stillborn in 2012. In a subsequent interview he said, 'It's something you accept that you are going to be dealing with for the rest of your life. In a strange way you don't want it to end because it's one of the few things that you have to remind you of the person who's not there.' I so agree with that sentiment. Some people may argue that holding on means you can never *move* on. Move on to where? My children have hinted that it would be OK if I wanted to meet someone – meaning another man – 'just as a friend.' I've got friends. 'Well, to take you out to eat.' I don't want to go out to noisy restaurants (see 'hearing aids'!). 'What about to the theatre, you enjoy that.' I'm quite happy to go on my own or with a girlfriend, thank you for your concern.

Would I want to 'meet someone else' – just as a friend or new partner? No thank you. Why, at my age, would I want to nurse another man through heart disease or cancer? Been there, done that. You never know, they say, he might need to look after you. Well maybe, I don't want to think about that.

The comedian, Ricky Gervais, voiced the same senti-ment in his wonderful series *After Life* on Netflix, which he wrote and directed. Playing the part of a man contem-plating suicide after the death of his beloved wife through sheer loneliness and depression, he is offended when his brother-in-law suggests he goes on a date. He says he still feels married to his wife and can't wait to be with her. Reminded that he doesn't believe in the afterlife, he says, 'I know – she's nowhere. But I'd rather be nowhere with her than somewhere without her.' With you there, mate.

Having said that, it does seem to be different for men as widowers. Men don't stay single for long. As long as they have a pulse and the requisite number of limbs, a new lady will appear on their arm within months. This is lovely for them. Nobody should be alone if they don't want to be and the length of time they take to form a new relationship has nothing to do with how much, or little, they loved their previous partner.

All I can say is, you need to look after yourself; eat sens-ibly, keep as healthy as possible so you don't cause problems for the people who love you, and don't do anything you don't want to do.

I have a Hindu friend who has described the beautiful rituals and traditions that take place during the initial mourning period after a death. Like most religions it focuses on family, friends and food. In the Jewish religion, when someone dies, the traditional greeting visitors offer to the mourners is, 'I wish you a "long life".' They may even add the rider: 'Please God to 120.' Well I don't know about you but I have no intention of living to 120, nor would I wish the same fate on anyone, so instead 'I wish you "love and laughter".' We're all in this together and we have a lot more living to do, so let's just get on with it.

I'd like to end this rather sad chapter on a lighter note. A few years ago, my friend Linda spotted the American comic Mel Brooks in a restaurant. This was just after his beautiful wife, the actress Anne Bancroft, had died and Linda went over to his table to commiserate.

'I know how you feel,' she told him, 'my mother passed away the same time as your wife.'
'I'm sorry to hear that,' said Mel, 'How old was she?'
'101,' replied Linda.
'Oh well,' said Mel, 'in that case, she was asking for it.'

10

AGE IS ONLY A NUMBER – NOT AN EXCUSE TO BE OLD

Talking of Mel Brooks, he was asked, at the age of 92, what was the secret of long life? He replied: 'Don't die'.

There was a life expectancy test in the newspaper recently, enabling you to determine how long you were going to live. I did it with my friend, Nancy. Apparently, the average age a woman lives to is 82, and you work out roughly when you are likely to pop your clogs by adding or subtracting years according to your lifestyle habits. For example, if you exercise three times a week you add seven years, and if you smoke you subtract ten years. If you eat broccoli every day you add five years, but if you drink a couple of glasses of wine with the meal you take off eight years, and so on. I lead quite a healthy life so I worked out that I can look forward to at least twenty years in a nursing home at £2,000 a week. Nancy discovered she died five years ago!

Research suggests that 68 is the age most people think 'old' begins. I think 75 is more to the mark but according to the popular press, 50 is the cut-off point of youth. We have all seen pictures of female stars of film or TV who have reached or – gasp! – gone beyond that advanced age.

Editors of 'women's pages' – who have barely finished teething and write the blurb accompanying these pictures – can't conceal their admiration that these aged goddesses are still able to walk unaided, let alone adopt a yoga pose!

Other, less talented 'celebrities', having reached the magic age of 50, feel compelled to bombard readers of newspapers with selfies of themselves in bikinis that show their bottoms. What are they actually saying here? 'Look at me, look at me, I'm 50 and my bottom is still at the top of my legs where it was when I was 49. Don't you just love me as much as I do?' Give it a rest, girls!

Old age creeps up slowly and usually without fanfare or acknowledgment. The realisation comes in waves; you can be watching a film and thinking, 'he's dead', 'she's dead' – 'Oh Lord, what's her name again?'

If you are in the 60-plus age group you are in good company as it is the fastest growing demographic of our time. Apparently, the average human life span gained more years during the twentieth century than in all prior millennia combined. Never before in history has the phase of later life had the potential to be so long and fruitful. Indeed, in 2020 there will be more people on earth over 65 than under five. That means more grandparents than grandchildren. How are we going to deal with this crucial demographic switch?

My maternal grandmother was over 90 when she died and, in those days, once their children were grown, she and her contemporaries struggled to make sense of a future in which their life's work was done, even though many of them remained healthy and capable of making further contributions to society (although not in grandma Katie's case, once the dreaded Alzheimer's took hold).

In the 1970s, a lot of women in their 30s and 40s went back to college which meant they broke out of the mould and redefined their roles. A friend of mine retrained as a barrister once her two children were safely ensconced in secondary school and said she was not the only older student sitting next to the 18-year-olds in the lecture hall; some of the other students were grandparents.

I loved that story about the French woman, Jeanne Calment, who became a global celebrity when she died in 1997 at the age of 122, holding the record as the world's oldest person. Only she wasn't. In fact, she was the *daughter* of Jeanne – Yvonne – who registered her mother's death as her own, then aged 34, and assumed her mother's identity to avoid paying crippling inheritance tax. Crafty, no? She managed to fool the world that she was Jeanne for the next six decades, despite being twenty-three years younger than her mother, and was actually 'only' 99 when she died.

My friends and I often wonder if we are turning into our mothers. As I mentioned earlier, my own mother was very fashion-conscious and was the most successful salesperson in Fortnum & Mason's fashion department for many years, with wealthy customers asking for her by name. She had a wonderful collection of beautiful hats which she adorned with flowers and ribbons, and which I didn't have the heart to give to a charity shop when she died. They are still at the top of my wardrobe and when my sister had to go to some fancy do, she came to borrow one. Sitting in front of the mirror with this hat on, we both gasped; it was as though our mother was sitting there! It left us both a bit shaky.

I'm certain I have inherited her critical nature, which, being aware of I try to temper, but she taught me how to be a good hostess and I owe her a debt of gratitude for encouraging me to do some exercise when I was so fat after baby number three. Her one action in dragging me along to the exercise class she attended in a dingy church hall eventually blossomed into my entire career.

When I voice my concern about familial dementia to a doctor or counsellor, they always say firmly, 'You are not your mother, it won't necessarily happen to you', but it doesn't exactly dispel my fears. I console myself by the fact that she took one of those old diazepam sleeping tablets every night from her 40s onwards, which have been proved to cause dementia, whereas I have never done that.

Everyone experiences old age differently and most of the people I know tend to be open to new ideas and new experiences, retaining the same deep sense of curiosity and discovery that they had as children. Some don't, however, and refuse to embrace even the simplest measures that would enhance their living conditions.

There was a lovely television series which ran for forty-four episodes in the 1970s and 80s called *Rumpole of the Bailey*. Do you remember that? It was written by John Mortimer and starred the actor Leo McKern as the grumpy barrister, Horace Rumpole, who was decidedly stuck in his ways. When told he should 'move with the times', he said, 'If I don't like the way the times are moving, I shall refuse to accompany them.' We all know people who think like that.

At least after a certain numbers of birthdays you only get one candle on your cake to blow out! And you begin to think differently: my sister went online to order her favourite deodorant. There were only two left so she hurriedly ordered them both. She thought the box she accepted from the delivery man was rather large for two deodorants and, upon opening it, discovered she had ordered two boxes of 12. Her first thought was, 'that should see me out!' This has become a recurring phrase with me and my friends whenever we buy a new purchase, from a kettle to an expensive handbag – that should see me out!

Most of us will spend a good twenty years or so in, hopefully, healthy active post-retirement, and sitting around doing nothing is hardly a realistic plan for happiness. You need to plan for old age and not simply financially, though of course that's important. There has to be a plan to stay involved in the community, with your family and spending time doing what you love. The most unhappy people in retirement are those who withdraw from involvements and expect people to come to them rather than reaching out, and who don't engage with family or discover new interests. As the writer, Diana Athill, said in her book, *Somewhere Towards the End* which she wrote in her 90s: 'The luckiest elderly people of all are those who have something in their own heads that they want to do such as writing or painting. That is a gift. If you don't have that gift you must look for it and find something that interests you.'

Research shows that the most important aspect of getting older is the need to continue giving to others. I know people who have been so impressed with the care shown to someone they love during their final weeks in a hospice that they feel the need to give something back, so they volunteer to serve in the shop or raise money to keep it going.

It's also important to speculate about your future in practical ways. It's never too early to start considering the basic questions: what sort of life do I want to live? Where and with whom? Am I going to stay in my present home or move to be nearer a family member? (Is that a threat,

Mum?) Do I want to travel? (Don't ask me to go with you!) Do I need to take out private health insurance? (Ask my son-in-law, Steve). All important points to ponder over to ensure a comfortable and interesting old age.

'Are You Lonesome Tonight?' – Elvis Presley

Answer: Probably. If you have lost a spouse, the loneliness sometimes hits you like a thump on the head. It's not there all the time because you have family and friends and hopefully, a job, occupation or group-based hobby to take your mind off it. But you can't expect those close to you to be mind readers when a rainy Sunday stretches ahead of you in endless empty hours.

You read about elderly people not speaking to a soul for days on end and it's very sad. If they are disabled and housebound then more effort should be made by the relevant councils to contact these people. But if you are able-bodied and still have your marbles, there is so much you can do to stave off loneliness. How would you feel about volunteering as a helper at your local hospital? Towards the end of 2018 the *Daily Mail* began a concerted campaign to recruit volunteers to join their NHS Hospital Helpforce. Every NHS hospital is short of nurses and auxiliary staff, and those that are there are really stretched to the limit. They just don't have time to sit with an elderly patient and listen to their stories, or feed those who have difficulty managing on their own. The Helpforce were looking for ordinary people, not necessarily with nursing experience, to pledge so many hours a week to put in the time at their local hospitals. Their duties could be anything from manning a desk directing patients to their relevant departments, playing or reading to children on the ward, making a cup of tea for visitors or pushing a trolley of snacks around the wards. It doesn't matter how old you are. My cousin, Colin, 84, is a welcomer at a huge hospital near his home. He retired from his accountancy firm several years ago and looked around for something to do after his wife, Mary, threatened to leave if he didn't stop rearranging her stacking of the dishwasher. His job, wearing his bright volunteer sash, is to greet people who enter and stand around looking lost. He then accompanies them through the endless corridors to their appointment, chatting reassuringly all the way.

Another key role is played by the discharge volunteers (not what you might think!) who offer support to the elderly – especially those aged 70 and over – leaving hospital to return to an empty home. The team at the hospital where Colin works has a budget of £10 per person and will pop to the shops and buy milk, bread and a meal to tide them over for the first few hours.

It's a brilliant idea and you need only put in as little as three hours a week if that's all you can spare. Nearly 30,000 people signed up during 2018 and not only does it free up the nurses to do their clinical work, but the satisfaction and actual buzz that the volunteers get from helping to run the NHS is immeasurable.

The *Daily Mail* campaign only lasted for a couple of months but if you get lonely sometimes and fancy doing something positive and life-enhancing like that, do contact your local hospital and see if you can join their army of volunteers. You'll be glad you did.

I asked around for other ways to combat loneliness and my neighbour, Jocelyn, said she only discovered she couldn't sing when she joined a choir! This did not deter her and obviously didn't bother the other participants in the group, as she demonstrated to me by singing her part of the Beach Boys song 'Good vibrations.' Oh dear God! But, as she informed me, researchers have found that levels of the natural brain compound anandamide, or AEA – dubbed the 'bliss molecule' – soared in women who were members of choirs and enhanced their mood. Apparently, they come out of rehearsals feeling energised, happy and buoyant. This prompted the researchers to claim that bursting into song could help those with depression or anxiety. Personally, I think it would have the reverse effect for anyone unfortunate enough to stand next to Jocelyn when she sings, but still!

Apart from choirs, there are many organisations to keep the old brain cells ticking over and make you feel part of the continuing spectrum of life. I have joined the University of Third Age (U3A) which recently opened a branch in my district. This is for older and retired people to broaden their minds and meet new people by joining a specific activity. There are dozens of courses such as learning bridge or a foreign language, psychology, yoga, art, theatre trips, and talks on every subject under the sun. It doesn't cost much to join, and you are bound to find something there to whet your interest as well as making a load of new friends.

How about a writing course, which features on every U3A timetable and which will help you construct a memoir of your life for your grandchildren? I bet, when you stop to think about it, you have lots of interesting stories you could tell. Google *University of Third Age* and see if there is a branch near you.

I also heard about an organisation that sounds like a lot of fun. It's called the Red Hat Society which started in

America and spread into many countries. It's for likeminded women to get together in local groups for activities like lunch or going to the theatre. Its aim is to 'connect, support and encourage women in their pursuit of fun, friendship, freedom, fulfilment and fitness while supporting members in the quest to get the most out of life.' The only rule is that every time you meet, women over 50 must wear a red hat and, if you are under 50, it's a pink hat. You can become a 'queen' and start your own group or join an existing one in your district. The pictures on their website show women all donned in a variety of hats having a great time.

I'm throwing these ideas out for you to explore if you want to. My advice is, don't just sit at home watching TV and making miniature wine glasses out of the foil wrappers of Quality Street chocolates. Get out and do something – anything – to retain the qualities that have made you the interesting person you are and always have been.

'I Remember You' – Frank Ifield

Or as Maurice Chevalier sang in the film *Gigi*, 'Ah I remember it well' – although today his character would be considered to be the sort of pervy old bloke who hangs around parks and primary schools! 'Thank heaven for little girls' – really?!!

When I used to visit my Auntie Sonia in her nursing home, I sometimes sat in on the reminiscence session where the carers sit with a group of dementia residents and encourage them to speak about their experiences of the past and what they remember. This is especially important to jog their memories and, hopefully, initiate a spark of recognition in the present day.

This took me back to my childhood days growing up in the 1940s. Are any of the following familiar to you?

- Sitting with my parents on a Friday evening watching a television magazine programme – the first of its kind – called *Kaleidoscope* with presenters, MacDonald Hobley and Ronnie Waldman.
- Rushing to finish my homework in time to listen to *Dick Barton, Special Agent*. Heaven forbid if I missed a daily episode, I wouldn't know what they were talking about at school!
- My first gramophone which needed to be wound up and a fresh needle inserted every time it played a vinyl record. Eddie Fisher singing *Downhearted* anyone?
- *The Goon Show* with Peter Sellers, Harry Secombe et al – which I pretended to find funny but was never really amused by people talking in silly voices.

Will I remember these things when I'm really, really old? I wonder. Which leads me to:

'Still Crazy After All These Years' – Paul Simon

In a previous chapter I outlined the best way to keep your brain healthy and delay any cognitive decline by doing mental puzzles and keeping physically fit, but suppose there was a simple blood test that could tell you whether you were genetically likely to develop dementia, would you take it? Actually there is, although I don't think it's a simple one: it's an APOE4 which would tell if you had the dementia gene and were therefore likely to inherit the disease. It's estimated that about five per cent of the population carry two copies of the E4 variant of the APOE gene, which makes them fifteen times more likely to develop Alzheimer's later in life.

My aforementioned Auntie Sonia had full-blown Alzheimer's so she obviously had the full whack of the E4 variant. She had no idea where she was, didn't recognise me or my sister – although she smiled at her and scowled at me – and had no real quality of life. She couldn't read a book or understand television programmes, although she liked the music channels with people dancing. Yet her heart was strong and she survived year after year in this state of being dressed, fed, taken to the loo, and put to bed by a series of patient and kindly carers.

My mother, Auntie Sonia's sister, had vascular dementia caused by little strokes in the brain, each one rendering her more and more helpless in looking after herself. She also ended up in a nursing home, as did her mother, my maternal grandmother, Katie. Uh-Oh! As I mentioned before, this does not bode well for me. I take after my mother's side of the family whereas my sister, Marilyn, is more like our father's family. As she says, bitterly, 'I inherited the bags under his eyes.' I have long pondered as to whether I should find out if I do have the dementia gene, but hesitate for a number of reasons; firstly, if the result were positive, it would be good to know as it would give me the nudge I need to get my affairs documented, and the mess which is my filing cabinet sorted to make life easier for my children once I succumb. Yet – and yet – would that mean that every time I accidently left my key in the front door or got momentarily stuck on a word that I might use all the time, cause me to think 'OK, here we go, it's starting'? Maybe it's better not to know.

Another test designed to spot dementia in its earliest stages is being developed to measure the intensity of blood flow travelling along the carotid arteries, which go up the sides of your neck taking blood to your brain. I'm too old for this test which needs to be carried out in your 40s or 50s, but this ultrasound scan can identify those at risk of cognitive decline in later life, particularly in relation to language and memory. If the carotid artery is healthy, it is elastic and flexible and the blood flows easily to the brain. But age and problems like high blood pressure and diabetes can stiffen the arterial walls affecting blood flow which eventually causes damage to the brain cells.

This test could be used to identify people at risk of heart disease and dementia who could benefit from preventative drugs. A spokesman from UCL's Institute of Cardiovascular Science said: 'Potentially, this could be a test to spot cognitive decline in middle-aged adults well in advance of actual symptoms.'

In the meantime, I suppose I could request to join a memory clinic, such as the one being conducted by Professor Peter Garrard at St George's Hospital in South London, for people worried about their mental health. He and his team use simple word tests to assess the breakdown in cognitive function – a term encompassing all mental abilities, such as reasoning and memory. Other tests rely on natural uses of speech such as narrative storytelling, everyday conversation or describing a simple act like making a cup of tea. The participants are invited back once a month to repeat the tests to check on their progress. There is also the state-of-the-art private Re:Cognition Health clinic off London's Harley Street, which is run by some of the country's leading brain and memory experts. A friend of mine was directed there by her doctor when she began showing enough symptoms to worry her family. Being slightly claustrophobic, she dreaded the thought of the tunnel-like 3T MRI scanner which she would have to go through to check whether her poor memory was caused by specific signs of brain shrinkage, or other abnormalities. A kindly nurse reassured her by asking which music she would like to help her relax whilst in the scanner. My friend opted for 'anything by Frank Sinatra.' She put the headphones on, closed her eyes and heard: 'And now the end is near, and I face the final curtain ...'!

At the time of writing it is estimated that there are around 850,000 people with dementia in the UK, costing the NHS £23 billion a year. That number is set to soar to two million by 2051. A staggering two-thirds of them are women and scientists have no idea why there is this disparity between the sexes. Although dementia is more likely to strike in later life, it is not an inevitable part of it. Around 17% of people over the age of 80 have it, but that means the other 83% do not. Hopefully, you and I are amongst that group. Studies of the risk factors suggest a severe bash on the head can increase the likelihood of developing it, but there's not a lot you can do about that. Lack of sleep is, apparently, another factor and it is well known that those with neurological degenerative diseases such as Alzheimer's sleep badly. So, what comes first? Does a lack of sleep cause deterioration in the brain or are those at high risk of Alzheimer's more likely to toss and turn at night? Scientists are conducting a study in the sleep laboratory at the University of East Anglia (UEA) to try and find the answer. Forty hapless volunteers are going to be divided into two groups and take part in sleep deprivation experiments to see how this effects performing everyday tasks, as well as challenging things such as memory, balance, coordination and focus. One group will be kept awake for forty hours and the others will be allowed short naps. That does not sound like much fun but, ultimately, this could help doctors identify whether specific problems with sleeping might identify dementia at an early stage. However, you can control all the usual stuff; smoking, obesity, diabetes, high blood pressure and high cholesterol, which are all associated with the onset of Alzheimer's. Currently there is research going on to see if drugs similar to statins, which lower cholesterol in the blood and dampen down artery inflammation, could also prevent inflammation in the brain which is linked to dementia. That's the good news.

The bad news: there is currently no cure for Alzheimer's and, although a raft of treatments can reduce the impact for a little while, once diagnosed the mental decline is inevitable. No drugs have yet been able to stop or reverse the proteins that damage the brain. I'm heartened by the findings reported by the Mayo Clinic which reviewed more than 1,600 papers on the subject of dementia and found 'very compelling' evidence that aerobic exercise, or any exercise that gets the heart pumping harder, can preserve cognitive abilities, reduce the risk of dementia and slow the condition's progression once it starts.

Yay – that's me sorted then! As a fitness instructor I still teach or go to other classes up to eight sessions a week, yet I still can't remember the name of that guy who presented the quiz game *Fifteen to One* which I used to watch with Mo in the afternoons. Can you? It's all a bit worrying. I've told the members of my exercise class to let me know if I suddenly start spouting rubbish during the lesson and one of them said 'How would we know the difference?' Nice!

On a serious note, there are thousands of people suffering from varying degrees of dementia who are isolated in their homes and relying on carers from social services to visit and maybe help to get them up and dressed and make sure there is food for the next meal. If you know of such a person, do tell them about Memory Cafes. These were started in the late 1990s by a Dutch psychiatrist, Dr Bere Miesen, who wondered what could be done about the stigma and neglect faced by those with dementia and their carers. He set up the first Memory Cafe and there are now thousands of them all over the world. They are popping up in pubs, churches, community centres and care homes often run by charities or church groups. All that's needed is a kettle, teabags and biscuits and they welcome dementia sufferers and their carers to come along and take part in quizzes, sing-alongs and simple word games. A friend who set one up in North London was surprised when it became a haven for lonely people as well. The basic pattern for them across the world remains remarkably consistent – love, care and activities offered in an informal environment. If you fancy setting up a Memory Café in your area, visit www.memcafe.org

'Fame / I'm Gonna Live Forever' – Irene Cara

Not if I can help it! I have no wish to live past the age of 90 – if I get that far. May I quickly state that I am in no way suicidal nor morbid. I am very happy currently being the age that I am, and I promised my husband that I would do my best to stick around to see the grandchildren safely grown up. But 90 is my cut-off point. By that time I will be ready to say, 'thank you very much, I've had a lovely life, I've been blessed with healthy children and grandchildren and it's now time for me to join my darling husband and friends in 'heaven' or wherever they are. Don't scoff; you don't know what you don't know!

How will I achieve this? I've no idea. I think that after the age of 80, most people's thoughts turn to an exit route and would rather opt for a quick and pain-free death any time soon than endure long drawn-out days being hoisted from bed to commode to wheelchair then back to bed again. Who doesn't dread that slow descent into senility? I tried to form a pact with my eldest grandson, who is in his early 20s, and said to him, 'Darling, can I rely on you to find a way to have me bumped off when I reach 90?' Wise head on young shoulders he replied, 'Why don't you wait till you get there and see how you feel then. You might change your mind.' Possibly, but I don't think so. I guess I could try the same time-honoured method I use when I want to wake up at a certain time. I'm sure you've done the same. Before dropping off to sleep I tell myself firmly, 'Wake up at 7.30 a.m.' and, even though I set the alarm as a precaution, I inevitably wake up just before it rings. Maybe I can do something similar here – 'Happy 90th birthday, Lee, now off you pop!' Although judging from my family history I'll probably be gaga by then and forget to do it!

There are countless articles in magazines and newspapers telling you how you can live to be 100 years old. As stated above, there is no cure for Alzheimer's or dementia so why would anyone in their right mind (ha ha) wish to live to 100? I don't get it. There is no one – and I stress, no one – who is in their 90s who hasn't got some sort of deterioration either in body or mind. Yes, you hear of the odd nonagenarian completing a marathon or climbing Mount Everest or winning a chess competition, but they are just freaky. The average person suffers from either mental deterioration or physical symptoms like arthritis, joint problems and digestive issues. The body wears out – fact. A letter from the Queen does not compensate for living in constant pain or with a head full of fog. As comic George Burns said, as he struggled to gather enough puff to blow out the century of candles on his birthday cake, 'If I knew I was going to live this long, I would have taken better care of myself!' Surely the point is not how long you live but how *well* you live, right up to the end.

Maybe my constant visits to Auntie Sonia in her nursing home had something to do with my mindset. She had no children of her own so Marilyn and I were her sole next-of-kin and responsible for her health and wellbeing. One of us popped in to visit her every day and each time my heart would sink. Seeing those unfortunate people sitting in rows in their wheelchairs, some of them slumped to one side having obviously suffered a stroke or others jabbering and crying with confusion at their surroundings, it was very upsetting. The carers were absolutely wonderful, I really can't praise these selfless people enough for what they have to deal with day in and day out, I know I couldn't. I would chat to them sometimes and they would point out a man looking blankly ahead with his hands encased in soft, fabric 'boxing' gloves to prevent him pulling out the feeding tube going into his stomach, or his catheter, and tell me he was once a famous lawyer. The lady with unkempt hair and her skirt riding up in an undignified way used to be a respected gynaecologist. I could weep for them. Please God, don't let me end up like that.

I'm sure *they* didn't want to either, but medical ethics seem to state that people must be kept alive at all costs. Although Auntie Sonia had a 'do not resuscitate' note in her file, at the slightest sign of infection she was prescribed antibiotics or ferried to hospital to be poked and prodded by medics struggling to find a suitable vein in her withered arm to insert an IV drip, while she screamed and cried in pain and confusion. All to prolong this miserable existence. Why?

I'm not going to go into the harrowing details of Auntie Sonia's final day on earth, aged 93, suffice to say that, against our wishes, paramedics were called and insisted on carting her off to hospital again even though she was obviously *in extremis*. Feisty to the end, Auntie Sonia chose to mount her own final little act of rebellion by dying in the ambulance en route to the hospital. This caused a huge delay in the issuing of the death certificate as the nursing home was in one district and the hospital in another and she died somewhere in between.

All this is why I – and I urgently suggest that *you* – make a proper living will. Not the old kind of advance directive where you fill in a vague form that the doctors, and probably your family who love you and want you around longer, will ignore, but a proper document registered with a firm of solicitors which is legally binding. This is so that while you still have the capacity to make decisions, you can issue specific instructions regarding your care in the event of a stroke or dementia preventing you from doing so in the future.

Doctors are trained and programmed to keep you alive regardless, although attitudes are softening towards desperately ill patients, such as those being kept alive on life-support machines. The British Medical Association

(BMA) has controversially agreed that doctors can ask these patient's relatives if there is any evidence in emails or messages on Facebook that would indicate whether the patient would prefer to die in those circumstances. This was branded 'ill-judged' by a group of doctors opposed to euthanasia and 'mercy killing' after a Supreme Court ruling in 2018 stated that doctors no longer needed to ask a judge for permission to remove food and liquid tubes keeping an incapacitated patient alive. The test case involved a 74-year-old woman who fell into a coma in hospital. Her daughter found an email from her mother stating that if she got dementia to 'get the pillow ready.' The High Court judge ruled that she could die based on her wishes expressed in the email.

After this ruling the BMA advised doctors to confer with the patient's family for permission to remove 'clinically-assisted nutrition and hydration' and should abide by their wishes in the event of there being no hope of a full recovery. This is progress of sorts but there is a difference between people in a coma and unlikely to recover, and someone with incurable cancer or dementia. Therefore, if you don't want to spend your last days with tubes coming out of every available vein or being jerked around on a bed at the mercy of a defibrillator, check out the following:

You need to download form LP1H which is the Lasting Power of Attorney for Health and Welfare, issued by the Office of the Public Guardian (OPG). This is a rather formidable twenty-page missive and you might need help filling it in, but please don't be put off by that as it's quite simple really. Even I figured it out and normally a veil comes down over my brain when faced with anything requiring more than my name and birth date.

If you get stuck, they offer an online guide for filling in each section so it's easy to follow. You start by appointing some people you trust and who know you well, like a close relative or your children. These are your 'attorneys' who will carry out your instructions if you are in a situation of being unable to speak for yourself. The OPG have taken the precaution of advising you to have 'replacement attorneys' as well in case your primary ones decide to emigrate to Australia in the meantime.

You need to choose your attorneys carefully as they are the ones who can give or refuse consent to life-sustaining treatment on your behalf. Remember, this is only if you are incapacitated and can't make these decisions for yourself. Life-sustaining treatment means care, surgery, medication or anything that's needed to keep you alive, for example: a serious operation, such as a heart bypass or organ transplant, cancer treatment or artificial nutrition or hydration – meaning those dreaded food tubes.

Whether some treatments are life-sustaining depends on the situation. If you had pneumonia, a simple course of antibiotics could be life-sustaining but if you were living with Alzheimer's, would you want to continue like that? That is for your chosen attorneys and the doctors to decide in conjunction with your wishes expressed in the Lasting Power of Attorney document. OK, serious stuff here: in my opinion, the most important section of the LP1H is page seven, where you document your specific instructions for your attorneys to follow should the situation arise. I have studied and researched this very carefully before putting pen to paper and advise you to do the same. I can tell you what I have put, but you might not agree with what I have written and must make your own decisions, bearing in mind I don't wish to go sailing on into my 90s even if I could still be teaching aerobics then!

Here is my declaration:
If I am diagnosed as being permanently mentally impaired with dementia or Alzheimer's disease, thereby being incapable of making my own decisions, I direct that my attorneys and others involved in my care withhold or withdraw treatment in accordance with my directions below:

- *If I have an incurable and irreversible terminal condition like cancer that will result in my death within a relatively short time.*
- *If I am diagnosed as persistently unconscious due to injury, disease or other means, and to a reasonable degree of medical certainty I will not regain consciousness.*
- *If I suffer a heart attack or a stroke.*
- *I not be given life support, cardiopulmonary resuscitation or any medical procedure, treatment or intervention which sustains, restores or supplants a spontaneous vital function.*
- *I not receive tube feeding including a nasogastric feeding tube, a percutaneous endoscopic gastrostomy (PEG) tube or a jejunostomy feeding tube, even if withholding such feeding would hasten my death.*
- *I not be given a tracheotomy or ventilator to assist breathing.*
- *In the event of an accident or cancer, I do not want a limb amputated.*

- *In the event of cancer, I not be given any form of chemotherapy or radiotherapy.*
- *If I should be in any of the above-mentioned conditions, and if my behaviour is violent or otherwise degrading, I want my symptoms to be controlled with appropriate drugs even if that would worsen my physical condition or shorten my life.*
- *If I should be in any of the above mentioned conditions and I appear to be in pain I want my symptoms to be controlled with appropriate drugs even if that would worsen my physical condition or shorten my life.*

This has to be signed and witnessed by an independent solicitor.

I bet you are now thinking 'bloody hell, that's a bit grim!' And you would be right. BUT I CAN CHOOSE TO REVERSE ANY OF THAT IF I'M STILL ABLE TO THINK AND MAKE DECISIONS FOR MYSELF. If I can't and I end up like Auntie Sonia, then those decisions stand.

After the final document is signed it is sent to the Office of the Public Guardian to be officially registered. Copies must be sent to everyone mentioned in the document and lodged with your solicitor and doctor's surgery. Job done. As Woody Allen said, 'It's not that I'm afraid to die, I just don't want to be there when it happens.' With you there, Woody.

There is another similar form dealing with your financial situation where you can list detailed instructions regarding who gets what in your will. I haven't done this one yet and I guess I'll have to get around to it someday. Meanwhile, my children can fight over who gets my extensive vinyl collection of soul and disco music from the 70s and 80s.

If you need any more information regarding these documents, do contact Age UK or go on their website.

I firmly believe in quality of life rather than longevity, but in the meantime I seem to be doing everything I can, unintentionally, to thwart my ambition to pop my trainers at 90. I have never smoked and don't like the taste of alcohol; I meditate every day for 20 minutes; I exercise every day as part of my job and choose food for health – most of the time. This fits in with advice given by scientists at North Western University in Chicago after many years of studying what they refer to as 'super-agers' – sprightly pensioners who are fit and healthy. Amongst other gems are to stay away from doctors if possible, as the need to find a cure for your minor ailment can escalate into numerous medications, most of which are to alleviate symptoms caused by the previous medications.

Just as I choose how I want to live, I really hope that one day the law will be changed to make assisted dying legal – not just for those who are terminally ill – but to ensure a sound of mind patient's wishes about their end of life care are sanctioned. I realise the subject of killing yourself by choice in old age is a subject no one, especially doctors, clergy and politicians, want to talk about. I described in the previous chapter how, if you have cancer, palliative care can improve your final months and allow you to lead a reasonably normal life free from pain and other debilitating symptoms. But suppose you reach a point, even when you're not ill, that you know in your heart and mind that it's time to go – that you *want* to go – then what? Tough! You jolly well stay alive until it's your rightful time. Why, as an intelligent, functioning being, can't I choose the time of my own death? I'm quite happy to sign a declaration saying I'm not being coerced into this by my wicked children who want all my money (what money?!) so what's the problem? The obvious objection would be if some unscrupulous grandson, desperately needing money for drugs, would persuade grandma to do away with herself, but this is *so* unlikely. We are not a nation of murderers! Why should this remote possibility condemn a large number of old people to living out their last few years in a manner not of their own choosing?

Of course, there must be stringent safeguards and surely every old person has someone they can trust even if it's a non-family member such as a neighbour. I'm not suggesting people keep a phial of diamorphine in the medicine cupboard along with the paracetamol, but in interviews with people who have signed up to an organisation like Dignitas or, as in certain American states, have been given the tools to commit suicide, they all say they won't necessarily use it but are relieved to know it's there should the day come. I know I have an ally in this: a lady called Susie Kennaway, aged 87 at the time of writing, whose son, Guy, has written a book about his feisty mother called *Time to Go* published in 2019. This is what she says: 'I am a woman who always stood up against things I considered to be wrong. In this case it is so utterly reasonable. I simply want to go while the going is still good. In light of the progress medicine has made, keeping a lot of us alive with a rotten quality of everyday living is senseless. I am not just speaking of illness and pain. I am talking about the time to live and the time to die, on behalf of those of us who do not want to end up in a care home. This is not about me. This is about a new campaign, a fight, I might say to the death and for the death. My wish is to go out at the top, dying as I myself will plan.'

Good on you, Susie! I'm with you all the way. And just to reassure her nearest and dearest she adds, 'but if it is the least bit of comfort to anyone, I can assure you the moment has not arrived.'

In the meantime, I might have to change my lifestyle in preparation for my eventual demise. So – can I cadge a cigarette off anyone? A spliff? Cocaine? Heroin? Midazolam? Whisky, gin? Anyone…?

'Keep Young and Beautiful' – Eddie Cantor

The song continues 'It's your duty to be beautiful' and ends with 'If you want to be loved.' Oh please! I guess that's how it was when that song was first recorded in 1933. A woman was expected to change her clothes and put on lipstick ready to greet her husband when he came home from work with a glass of whisky, his slippers and the aroma of a delicious meal cooking in the oven. Today's scenario would more likely be the wife frantically texting her partner at 5.00 p.m. instructing him to pick up some food on his way home and start the dinner because she has a conference call in ten minutes and will be late. Oh, and to collect the dry cleaning on his way.

Yes, fings ain't what they used to be, but it is what it is. We're still standing – well, most of us older folk – and we battle on the best we can. Having friends from multiple generations can help head off the loneliness that can ensue when your neighbours downsize from the family house to a flat, your friends die, or remarry and get absorbed into their new husband's life. Milestones, birthdays and the news that your 'little' 6ft 4in grandson is now driving a car (how did that happen?!) are constant reminders of the passage of time but you should not lose focus on finding meaning and quality in life. This means looking after yourself, eating healthily, exercising and keeping abreast of what is happening in the world.

'You Make Me Feel So Young' – Frank Sinatra

Think of an age – any number you like between 20 and 80 – when you felt good about yourself. When the stunning model Christie Brinkley turned 65, she said she felt so much younger and coined the phrase 'spirit age' – the age at which she thought of herself. Think back. What is *your* spirit age? This is the time when you actually felt young and, judging by the flirty compliments you were getting from people you mixed with either at work or socially, quite attractive. My spirit age is 32. I don't know why that number sticks in my mind; I guess my children were all at school then and after dropping them off I would hop on the tube to the (now sadly defunct) Dance Centre in London's Covent Garden to do Arlene Phillips's jazz class. (Remember me, Arlene – near the back by the window?) I felt strong and fit and I suppose I quite liked myself at that age. That is the age at which I am mentally stuck – although of course the mirror tells a different story – and I try and behave as if I were actually that age, with modifications of course.

Decide on your spirit age. Imagine yourself being young, slim and fit but with the added knowledge and intelligence you have accumulated over the years. If you do this, you will be thought of as forever young. This is important because we all have to try and counter social and cultural myths about what it means to be old. Avoiding conversations about how ignorant you are about modern life even if, like me, you still think Twitter is what birds do and you don't dabble in Facebook or Instagram. Advances in technology have accelerated the stereotype that old people can't keep up. You need to stay 'woke.' (Impressed, kids?!)

Also avoid joining in conversations that I call 'competitive ailments' – you know what I mean: one person starts the ball rolling by imparting bad news about someone they know who has contracted some terrible disease. Another will pipe up along the lines of 'you think that's bad, what about…' and someone else will come up with an even more gruesome tale of woe. The historian, Eric Hobsbawm used to describe these sorts of conversations as 'organ recitals.' Don't get sucked in.

To counter that, it's good to have a fund of humorous stories or funny incidents to relate when you're invited somewhere. I think it's important to be a good guest and join in by stating your views and opinions even if the youngsters roll their eyes and groan. Having said that, you have learned that you don't always have to be *right* – even when you are! Sometimes you let the other person win just to keep the peace and let them feel good. *You* know what makes life work; *they* will have to learn for themselves.

The main thing is to recognise what is important: love, family and relaxing with good friends that you've known for forty or fifty years and not worrying how you appear to them. This is the upside of being old – the fun, companionship, shared traits and easy camaraderie. They know and accept your faults, peculiarities, children, and share worries about grandchildren and state of the country and the world. While most people enjoy relative continuity over the decades, being able to adapt to the changing context of our lives is the key to success throughout life. The future is scary. Artificial intelligence will, we're told, destroy not just manual labour but professional jobs like accountants, solicitors, doctors and dentists. Robot gynae check anyone? 'Lie. Back. Place. Feet. In. The. Stirrups.' Nooooo!

I loved the story of the Japanese hotel run entirely by robots where one guest was woken every few minutes during the night by his personal robot repeating, 'I don't understand the question' – in response to his snoring! The hotel had to close down in the end because all the robots carrying the luggage up to the rooms and pushing the food trolleys kept crashing into each other and falling over, and the guests complained that there was no one to complain to!

I'm too nervous about having one of those computer pods like Alexa or Siri skulking in the corner of my living room. I actually don't find it too arduous a task to turn off a light or TV without shouting 'Alexa, turn the light off.' I would always say 'please' thereby eliciting a response 'You're welcome' and initiating a conversation which would mean I'd never get to bed! I'm also nervous it might be listening to everything I say and gathering information on my likes and dislikes to report back to some global corporation.

I can't picture a driverless car. Will it have a built-in nagging voice saying 'I said *left*, now you've missed the turning, mind that pothole, can we have different music please' just to be more authentic? Will our homes really be built using 3D printing and will armies of robots fight our wars?

Medical advances will probably be able to build spare parts for every organ and limb in the body – except the brain. So there will be millions of able-bodied people walking around, but not knowing who they are or where they're going.

But hey, whatcha gonna do? We'll just have to let those confident know-it-all youngsters sort it out while we sit back and relax. What are we watching tonight? I love *Greenleaf* on Netflix.

Oh – it was William G. Stewart – the man who presented *Fifteen to One*.

Phew!

ACKNOWLEDGEMENTS

When my scribbles took on the semblance of a book, I sent it to the wonderful **Wanda Whiteley** at Manuscript Doctor for appraisal, fully expecting her to say 'Bin it'. She didn't. Instead she pointed out where I was going wrong and, surprisingly, where I was going right.

This encouraged me to send it to **Richard Charkin**, saying I was looking for a Mensch (Hebrew definition: a person of integrity and honour) to publish my book. I really liked the Mensch publishing ethics, and explained what I wanted to achieve in my book which was to dispel the idea that older people were frail, dim-witted and a burden on society. Richard agreed that the message should be 'out there' and said he would publish my book. Thank you, Richard, you are a true Mensch.

I could not have got this far without the help of my brilliant daughter, **Sharon Pink** who took my garbled chapter summary and formatted it into a book proposal that no Mensch could turn down. Thank you, my lovely girl, for your infinite patience in dealing with my daily whingeing inability to master even the simplest computer manoeuvre and your staunch support in everything I do.

Once the contract was signed a number of the most talented people appeared in my inbox:

Miranda Vaughan Jones. I am most grateful to you for taking on the massive task of correcting my grammar and tightening up my ramblings into some coherent form, as well as curbing my propensity for endless lists. 'Choose three!' you ordered. I chose four. Thank you so much for your patience and for not getting irritated when I kept adding bits of text. You were so kind and we got there in the end.

Phillip Beresford. You blew me away with your inventiveness for the book cover! Sheer genius. I'm glad we found the picture of the little boxing figure taken by my photographer daughter, **Carolyn Djanogly,** who also took the lovely photo of her daddy and me.

Ruth Killick. Thank you so much for taking on the arduous task of getting this book out there. I know how difficult this is and I have been so impressed with your dedication and persistence. You have done a superb job.

In fact, thank you to everyone who has worked so hard to get this book onto the shelves. I thought books just magically appeared in bookshops, and certainly didn't appreciate how much effort went into their production. I think you're all amazing.

NOTE ON THE AUTHOR

Lee Janogly trained as a dancer in the 1960s with chore-ographer Arlene Phillips at the Dance Centre in Covent Garden, later qualifying as a fitness instructor. She opened her own exercise studio All That Jazz in North London in the 1980s, featuring classes in everything from Aerobics to Yoga.

After studying nutrition for many years, in the 90s Lee qualified as a diet counsellor with Nutrisystem. She subse-quently branched out on her own to combine diet coaching with customised exercise and still delivers her extended Living Slim Course for private clients.

Lee's first book *Stop Bingeing!* was published in 2000, followed by her second, *Only Fat People Skip Breakfast* in 2005. Her focus has always been to make reading about diet and fitness enjoyable and fun as well as inspiring.

Lee has appeared on TV and radio programmes, including ITV's Loose Women, Larry Grayson's Generation Game, LBC, BBC Radio London and other regional stations across the country, sharing her irreverent observations and answering listeners' questions.

Lee also provided in-flight exercise information for airlines. Even 35,000 ft in the air you can't escape her advice! Lee has five children and seven grandchildren and lives in North London. She still teaches up to eight sessions of exer-cise a week and, in her new book, has turned her attention to telling it like it is about getting old.

NOTE ON THE TYPE

The text of this book is set in Linotype Sabon, a typeface named after the type founder, Jacques Sabon. It was designed by Jan Tschichold and jointly developed by Linotype, Monotype and Stempel in response to a need for a typeface to be available in identical form for mechanical hot metal composition and hand composition using foundry type.

Tschichold based his design for Sabon roman on a font engraved by Garamond, and Sabon italic on a font by Granjon. It was first used in 1966 and has proved an enduring modern classic.